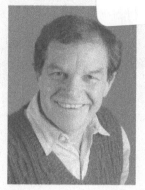

David Isaacs is a consultant paediatrician at the Children's Hospital at Westmead, in Sydney, and Clinical Professor in Paediatric Infectious Diseases at the University of Sydney. He has been a member of all of Australia's national immunisation advisory committees for the last 25 years. David has a passion for bioethics, and has published and taught extensively on ethical aspects of immunisation.

Defeating the Ministers of Death

The compelling history of vaccination

DAVID ISAACS

HarperCollins*Publishers*

HarperCollins*Publishers*

First published in Australia in 2019
by HarperCollins*Publishers* Australia Pty Limited
ABN 36 009 913 517
harpercollins.com.au

HarperCollins*Publishers*
Level 13, 201 Elizabeth Street, Sydney NSW 2000
Unit D1, 63 Apollo Drive, Rosedale, Auckland 0632, New Zealand
A 53, Sector 57, Noida, UP, India
1 London Bridge Street, London, SE1 9GF, United Kingdom
Bay Adelaide Centre, East Tower, 22 Adelaide Street West, 41st floor, Toronto,
   Ontario M5H 4E3, Canada
195 Broadway, New York NY 10007, USA

A catalogue record for this book is available from the National Library of Australia.

ISBN: 978 14607 5684 3 (paperback)
ISBN: 978 14607 1064 7 (ebook)

Cover design by Mark Campbell, HarperCollins Design Studio
Front cover image: *Lymphangioma circumscriptum* affecting the skin under the eye,
St Bartholomew's Hospital Archives & Museum, Wellcome Collection
Spine image: Illustration of face diseased with syphilis, Wellcome Collection
Back cover image: Hypodermic syringes, manufacturer's catalogue, p. 321, Wellcome Collection
Typeset in Sabon LT by Kirby Jones
Printed and bound in Australia by McPherson's Printing Group
The papers used by HarperCollins in the manufacture of this book are a natural, recyclable product made from wood grown in sustainable plantation forests. The fibre source and manufacturing processes meet recognised international environmental standards, and carry certification.

To Carmel

CONTENTS

Introduction

Recently I met a young couple whose six-week-old son had just died from whooping cough (pertussis). They were devastated, but they were also angry.

Their son had been too young for immunisation, but had caught whooping cough from a school-age sibling. The older child had been immunised, but whooping cough had been circulating among unimmunised children at school.

Why had the other parents not had *their* children immunised? How could they have been so selfish? Shouldn't there be a law against it?

Immunisation is a topic that polarises opinion. As with climate change, people either tend to trust the experts or doubt them, and there is little room for a halfway position. Ethicists wring their hands: people claim rights, yet rights conflict. One parent's right to decide whether or not their child is immunised can clash with another parent's right for their child to be protected from other children's infections.

There have always been opponents of immunisation. After immunisation was introduced at the beginning of the 19th century, there were large demonstrations in Britain and the United States. At one protest in Leicester, more than 80,000 people marched through the streets. The American opposition was also fierce, but more litigious.

Today, however, scientists can point to the remarkable successes achieved through immunisation. For centuries, smallpox was a devastating disease that killed many and permanently scarred survivors – the English historian Lord Macaulay called it 'the most terrible of all the ministers of death'. Even in 1950, the year I was born, an estimated 50 million people, about 2% of the world's population, still caught smallpox each year, and as many as 10 million of them died from it. By 1978, however, smallpox had been eradicated by immunisation: a remarkable achievement that shows the extraordinary potential of immunisation to save lives. Today there is almost no one alive who has seen a case of smallpox.

Travelling in Africa or Asia, you will still see people crippled by polio. Yet polio too will soon disappear. In 1988, there were 350,000 cases worldwide; in 2017 there were just 29.

Of course there is much still to be done. In Africa, I have seen babies and children racked with spasms from tetanus. I have watched helpless as an African doctor's 14-year-old son lapsed into a coma and died from rabies. I have seen hundreds of children die from meningococcal meningitis. I have seen wards of children with severe measles which, if they survived, left them weakened and vulnerable to dying from other infections such as severe gastroenteritis. Even in the United Kingdom and Australia, in years gone by, I saw children die or become brain-damaged from infections that have since all but disappeared due to immunisation programs.

The history of the development of vaccines by great scientists and doctors is one full of human interest, drama and magic. Of course, great scientists such as Louis Pasteur were flawed, like all humans, but that only adds to their intrigue. And this book aims to explore that human dimension: the people who developed the first vaccines; the children who were their first patients; those killed for trying to prevent polio. I will celebrate the successful control of many previously fatal infections, but also mourn those who died when early immunisation programs went wrong. And I will explore ethical issues, as well as the safety and effectiveness of vaccines.

People have written books about immunisation before. I wrote one in the year 2000 with the late lamented immunologist Gordon Ada called *Vaccination: The Facts, the Fears, the Future*. But in *Defeating the Ministers of Death*, my ambition is to inspire you by telling you the most exciting stories behind immunisation, and show you what these most human of stories have to teach us about ourselves.

CHAPTER 1

Our deadliest foes

The finely dressed crowd gathered in the White House was hushed. People were on tenterhooks and spoke in whispers. The orchestra too was silent; President Abraham Lincoln had forbidden any dancing.

Eleven years earlier, in 1851, the president's second child, Eddie, had died aged three after a harrowing seven-week illness of coughing fits and fevers, probably diphtheria or tuberculosis. Now two of the Lincolns' surviving sons, Willie and Tad, had caught typhoid, and lay weak with headaches, fevers, diarrhoea and severe aches and pains. Tad was recovering, but 11-year-old Willie was fading fast.

Mary Lincoln kept leaving the party, hurrying upstairs in her long white satin dress to be with her dying son. Mary's seamstress, ex-slave Elizabeth Keckley, later wrote about Willie's debilitating illness: 'The days dragged wearily by, and he grew weaker and more shadow-like. He was his mother's favourite child.'

When Willie finally died on 20 February 1862, Abraham Lincoln could scarcely believe it. He walked down the corridor to the room of his secretary John Nicolay and sobbed: 'Well, Nicolay, my boy is gone – he is actually gone!'

Willie's body was laid out in the White House on a huge rosewood bed, now called the Lincoln Bed. Elizabeth Keckley recorded the president's words: 'My poor boy, he was too good for this earth. God has called him home. I know that he is much better off in heaven, but then we loved him so much. It is hard, hard to have him die!' Then Lincoln buried his head in his hands and wept.

At the funeral, the Lincoln family gathered round the coffin to say farewell to Willie. Benjamin French, the funeral supervisor, wrote: 'While they were thus engaged there came one of the heaviest storms of rain and wind that has visited this city for years, and the terrible storm without seemed almost in unison with the storm of grief within.'

Willie's death rocked the Lincoln family to its core. For months afterwards, Abraham Lincoln would often retreat to a secluded room to weep. Mary was even more bereft. Elizabeth Keckley described her as 'an altered woman ... she never crossed the threshold of the Guest's Room in which he died, or the Green Room in which he was embalmed'. Abraham had to hire a nurse to look after her.

Yet Mary Lincoln's grief was only just beginning. One day in 1865, Abraham told Mary, 'We must both be more cheerful in the future. Between the war and the loss of our darling Willie we have been very miserable.' They went to the theatre that same evening. Suddenly a well-known actor, John Wilkes Booth, burst into their private box and unaccountably shot Abraham Lincoln in the back of the head. Six years later, Tad died aged 18 from heart failure, possibly caused by tuberculosis.

Abraham Lincoln will be forever remembered, and rightly so, as the Great Emancipator who won the American Civil War and set his country on the path to the abolition of slavery. But his tragic family history illustrates the precariousness of children's lives in that era. Only one of the Lincolns' four children – their eldest son Robert – lived to adult life. Nowadays they would all have survived, thanks to a combination of vaccines, antibiotics and improved sanitation.

Under attack

Nature is the world's greatest terrorist. While we may fear human terrorist attacks, in truth humans have always had far more to fear from infections.

In the fifth century BC, Athens and Sparta, the two most powerful city-states in Greece, became engaged in the bitter Peloponnesian War, which lasted 27 years. Athens lost the war, and this loss transformed ancient Greece, which became ravaged by vicious civil conflicts. Athens might well have won the war had it not been for a 'plague' in 430 BC, the second year of the war, that killed over 30,000 Athenians, many of them previously healthy young men and women. The historian Thucydides caught the plague and survived, so his descriptions of the suffering are particularly poignant:

> People in good health were all of a sudden attacked by
> violent heats ... the throat or tongue, becoming bloody and
> emitting an unnatural and fetid breath ... Discharges of bile

of every kind named by physicians ensued, accompanied by
very great distress ...

The body was ... reddish, livid, and breaking out into
small pustules and ulcers ...

The miserable feeling of not being able to rest or sleep
never ceased to torment them.

If the disease descended further into the bowels, inducing
a violent ulceration there accompanied by severe diarrhoea,
this brought on a weakness which was generally fatal.

Modern tests on teeth from an ancient Greek burial pit suggest
the so-called 'Plague of Athens' was actually typhoid fever,
although some experts dispute the validity of these tests.

Typhoid has all but disappeared from industrialised countries
because of improved sanitation and the provision of safe drinking
water. Modern wars bring their own horrors, but today a plague
of typhoid would be prevented by better hygiene, or the sick
would be cured with antibiotics. Children and young adults in
resource-rich countries are far less likely to die from infections
nowadays, though in many poor countries they remain at risk
(albeit far less risk than in ancient Greece).

The global rise in life expectancy is partly due to antibiotics
and improved living conditions. But it would not have been
possible without immunisation.

Sources of infection

Humans can become infected by bacteria, fungi or viruses.
Bacteria are micro-organisms that live almost everywhere on
Earth, including in and on our bodies. Most do us no harm, but

some cause infectious diseases, including tuberculosis, cholera and bubonic plague. Bacterial infections can often be cured with antibiotics. As well as mushrooms and toadstools, fungi include micro-organisms such as yeasts and moulds. Fungal infections are often of the skin, for example tinea, or of the lining of the mouth or vagina, as with thrush. But they can be more serious and invade the lungs or brain if the patient's immunity is very low. We use antifungal agents to treat fungal infections.

The word 'virus' derives from an ancient word common to Sanskrit, Greek and Latin meaning poison, and came to refer to snake venom in Middle English. The word 'virulent' has the same derivation. Unlike bacteria and fungi, viruses are not even alive; they are germs that reproduce by infecting a living cell, hijacking its genetic material and forcing it to make more viruses. Each virus contains only a handful of genes. The influenza virus has eight genes and HIV (the human immunodeficiency virus) has nine, whereas a human has about 20,000.

Small size is no hindrance, however, and viruses are the most common infections: children aged one to five have an average of more than six viral infections a year, mainly coughs and colds caused by respiratory viruses and diarrhoea (gastro) caused by gut viruses. There are just a few antiviral medicines, for example to treat herpes simplex and chickenpox viruses. Antibiotics have no effect on viruses whatsoever. A doctor may give them to a patient with a cough or bad cold, but this is just in case the cause is a bacterial infection.

More dangerous viruses can kill millions of humans. The British biologist and Nobel laureate Peter Medawar described a virus as 'a piece of nucleic acid surrounded by bad news'. From the 16th century onwards, viral infections like measles and smallpox introduced by European colonisation of the Americas killed over 90% of the indigenous population, immeasurably more than were killed by weapons. Smallpox killed 300 million people in the 20th century before it was eradicated by immunisation. Infectious diseases always have been and always will be a natural part of the human condition.

The notorious 'Spanish influenza' pandemic, which started in 1918 near the end of World War I and lasted for three years, infected 500 million people and killed more than 50 million people, many of them young, previously healthy adults. In *Pale Rider*, Laura Spinney writes that the 1918 influenza pandemic 'resculpted human populations more radically than anything since the Black Death'. Spinney took the name of her book from a short story called *Pale Horse, Pale Rider* by the United States writer and political activist Katherine Anne Porter, who almost died from influenza in Denver in 1918, aged 28. Her rich black hair fell out, grew back white and remained white until she died aged 90. The influenza killed young and old, rich and poor, from Alaska to Brazil to Odessa to South Africa to Zanzibar. The three-year pandemic killed far more people than died from warfare in both world wars combined.

It is not known where the influenza pandemic started; unproven theories include the over-crowded French trenches and even China. The poor Spanish were innocent: influenza spread from France to Spain during the war. The influenza was introduced into the United States by sailors arriving in Boston in August 1918. Within six months, over half a million Americans had died from the flu.

The government was desperate to study the virus with the aim of developing a vaccine. A thousand sailors imprisoned on Deer

Island in Boston Harbor for crimes such as desertion, drunkenness and delinquency were ordered to gather on the parade ground. A public health physician, Dr Joseph Goldberger, asked the men if they would volunteer to be infected with influenza. He told them what it would entail.

First a culture of influenza would be sprayed into their nostrils. If that did not cause them to catch the flu, they would be injected with suspensions of lung tissue (tissue shaken up with saline until dissolved sufficiently to be injected) from people who had died of the illness. Next they would have mucus from influenza patients sprayed into their eyes and noses and rubbed onto their throats. Finally each volunteer would have a seriously ill influenza patient cough straight into his face. The upside was that they would be pardoned if they survived.

Three hundred prisoners volunteered. Goldberger selected 62, and they were taken to a quarantine station and subjected to this battery of attempts to infect them.

At the end of the experiment they were all pardoned. Not one prisoner had caught influenza. Probably they had already been infected with influenza when the epidemic first hit Boston and were immune.

One person did catch influenza during the study: the doctor from the quarantine station who performed the experiments. He promptly died.

A disturbing feature of the pandemic was that it killed young healthy adults, whereas most influenza strains cause fatalities among the elderly. Many scientists tried to find the source of the 1918 influenza virus. One unsuccessful attempt involved looking for antibodies in blood from people living on remote islands who had survived the 1918 pandemic and never been infected with influenza since. Finally, in 2005, United States scientists were able to determine the genetic make-up of the pandemic influenza virus, with samples taken from the body of a woman who had died in 1918 and been buried in permafrost in Alaska, thus preserving her tissues for posterity. The virus was then reconstructed. When it was subsequently given to macaque monkeys, they mounted a vigorous immune response, known as a 'cytokine storm', and some died. This led researchers to conclude that many young adults died from pandemic influenza because the virus induced just such an overactive host response. It's tragic that so many young men and women were killed by their own immune system. The only possible solution would have been prevention, and by that I mean immunisation.

How infections occur

To understand how immunisation works, we first need to understand what infections are and how humans respond to them. Humans evolved after micro-organisms, and to a certain extent we have always competed with each other for survival. This is often portrayed using military language: a 'war on infection'. But, as with the war on cancer, or indeed the War on Terror, to simplify the enemy is to underestimate the problem and risk missing the subtleties. The relationship between humans and infection is more complex than a war, although to this day when war breaks out infectious diseases soon follow.

A human infection is sometimes said to occur when a micro-organism 'invades' the body and causes disease. The womb contains no micro-organisms, and almost all newborns are completely sterile when they are born. Within a matter of hours after birth, the baby has acquired micro-organisms from the environment all over its skin and different micro-organisms throughout its gut or intestinal tract. These micro-organisms do not kill the baby because they do not invade. They do not invade because most of them are not very *virulent* (warlike), and because the baby already has an immune system that recognises and deals with those organisms that can be *pathogenic* (cause disease). Our immune system is highly complex. It can recognise and destroy most foreign agents – not just micro-organisms like viruses and bacteria, but also cancer cells.

It makes no sense, thinking strictly in terms of survival of the fittest, for a micro-organism to kill the host on which its own survival depends. What is in the micro-organism's best interests is to live in harmony with its human host. For example, a respiratory organism like the pneumococcus – named because it can cause pneumonia – would be better off lazing in a warm bath of nasal mucus and reproducing from time to time than it would invading the lungs.

Indeed, most of the time the former is exactly what the pneumococcus does, lucky thing, in a process we call colonisation. Colonisation allows the organism to live in equilibrium with the host. We call this existence a commensal relationship: when the micro-organism benefits and the host is not harmed. If the host also benefits, it is a symbiotic relationship, while if the host is harmed the organism is a parasite.

Only occasionally does the pneumococcus spread to the lungs to cause pneumonia, or via the bloodstream to cause meningitis. If that kills the host, the pneumococcus also dies.

'Why did *my* child get that infection?' parents of seriously infected children often ask. Why indeed? Infectious disease doctors teach that an infection occurs as a result of three main factors.

The first is the host. The host may be particularly susceptible to infection: infections are more common in very young babies and the very elderly because the immune system works less efficiently at the extremes of life. Infections are also more common and more severe in 'immunocompromised' people – those whose immune systems are weakened by certain drugs, by pregnancy, or even by other infections, such as HIV infection.

The second factor is the organism: some organisms are far more virulent than others. People almost never die from being infected with the common cold virus but almost never recover from rabies virus infection.

The third factor is the environment: you cannot catch malaria without being bitten by a mosquito; you cannot catch tuberculosis without being coughed on by someone with pulmonary tuberculosis or without drinking tuberculosis-infected milk; and you are more likely to develop pneumococcal pneumonia if you or your parents smoke. We cannot always answer the question 'Why did my child get that infection?', but when we can, we usually find the infection is due to interactions between two or three of these factors.

Knowing the reasons people catch infections helps us prevent them. We can influence the environment, for example through improved sanitation and cleaner air, to try to prevent exposure to organisms. We can destroy the organisms causing bacterial infections with antibiotics. We can also influence the host. It is a truism that prevention is better than cure, but arguably our most powerful tool is the use of immunisation to educate the host's immune system and prevent infections.

How immunisation works

Writing about the Plague of Athens, Thucydides observed:

> Yet it was with those who had recovered from the disease
> that the sick and the dying found most compassion. These
> knew what it was from experience, and had now no fear for
> themselves; for the same man was never attacked twice –
> never at least fatally.

Thucydides had recognised two important things: firstly people who had been infected were much less likely to catch the infection again, and secondly if they did get re-infected, the infection was less severe. We would express the first observation as the concept of *immunity* to infection, and the second as the concept that the immune system can reduce the *severity* of re-infection.

The reason children who have had measles do not get it a second time is that their immune system remembers the measles virus for the rest of their life. If they are exposed to measles virus again, even as an adult, their immune system destroys the virus before it can reinfect them. There are some infections we can catch a second time as our immunity wanes – for example, respiratory syncytial virus (RSV) infection, which can give infants a nasty lung condition – but repeat infections are less severe because the immune system remembers and kicks in.

Immunisation works by taking an organism, modifying it so that it is less virulent, then giving the modified organism to a person to stimulate their immune system. Vaccines can either prevent infections or make them less severe. Measles vaccine protects over 95% of people immunised against infection.

Chickenpox vaccine is only 80 to 85% effective in preventing infection, but immunised children who do catch chickenpox have a much milder infection than unimmunised ones, with fewer spots, less fever and far fewer complications.

People sometimes get confused between immunisation and vaccination. Vaccination refers to the physical process of giving a vaccine. Immunisation refers to the way a vaccine stimulates a person's immune response to provide protection against infection. But since the whole point of giving a vaccine is to induce an immune response, there may be little point in maintaining the distinction, and many of us use the two words interchangeably. When we immunise we are stimulating a specific immune response, meaning the immune system learns to protect against that particular organism but not against other unrelated organisms.

Another important concept is herd immunity: immunising a proportion of the population gives some protection against the disease to unimmunised people. The term was first used in 1923, and derives from the concept of a herd of buffalo that form a circle, with the strong on the outside protecting the weak on the inside. Other terms for herd immunity include 'population immunity' and 'community immunity', a term that rhymes but has little else to commend it.

If there is a large outbreak of, say, measles, once almost everyone has been infected, they are immune and the disease stops circulating. At this point, even susceptible children do not get infected. This is natural herd immunity.

There are some people who doubt the existence of vaccine-induced herd immunity. However, there is clear evidence that it occurs, although its extent varies from disease to disease, depending on how infectious the disease is and how protective the vaccine. Tetanus immunisation only protects the person immunised, and provides no herd immunity whatsoever, because there is no person-to-person spread and the responsible organism comes not from humans but from the soil.

In contrast, schoolchildren but not the elderly were routinely immunised against influenza in Japan for 25 years from 1962 to 1987, yet rates of influenza among the elderly were low. When Japan stopped immunising schoolchildren against influenza, rates of influenza in the elderly rose three- or four-fold. When school-based immunisation was reintroduced, influenza rates in the elderly fell again. The clear implication is that influenza circulates in schoolchildren, who can infect the elderly; immunising schoolchildren against influenza thus also protects the unimmunised elderly. This is a classic example of vaccine-induced herd immunity.

The concept has been likened to 'the tragedy of the commons', a term first used in 1833 by the English economist William Forster Lloyd in a lecture he published about population control. Lloyd used the analogy of farmers whose cattle share pasture on common land. If all the farmers behave responsibly in terms of the number of cattle they put on the commons, there is enough pasture to go round and all the cattle thrive. If one selfish farmer puts extra cattle on the land, the amount of pasture may suffice, but if *every* commoner adds extra cattle, the pasture will be consumed and all the cattle will starve.

In 1969, ecologist Garrett Hardin used Lloyd's analogy to discuss ecological problems such as overfishing the oceans. The idea has since been expanded to other situations, including immunisation. If lots of people stop immunising their children against measles, say, then the disease will return with a vengeance and cause outbreaks.

Dangerous complacency

Armed with this knowledge about immunisation, we are in a better position to reassure people who have misgivings about vaccines. People are understandably cautious, if not downright suspicious, about having their children injected with foreign proteins. Yet each of us when healthy carries around at least as many bacteria and other non-human cells as we have human cells. We live our entire lives in peaceful coexistence with billions of foreign organisms, which benefit us more than they attack us. The foreignness of vaccines is nothing compared with the foreignness of the organisms we all carry on and inside us.

The vaccines we use for immunisation stimulate the host's natural immune system, so are not totally unnatural, even if they do manipulate nature to protect humans from infection. But we manipulate nature in many ways. We use fertilisers to increase the yield of crops. We build dams to divert rivers and bridges. We manufacture cars and trains and planes to travel. To call vaccines foreign and unnatural is a fairly weak argument for not using them.

Some immunisation sceptics say that infections result primarily from malnutrition. They argue that if people receive the correct nutrition, vaccines are unnecessary. Malnutrition certainly increases the risk of infection – and for many infections nowadays there is a poverty gradient, with a greater incidence and severity in low-income countries and among the poor in industrialised countries. But there are many other important factors that determine who will catch an infection.

Sanitation is one of the most important influences on enteric diseases – diseases of the gut that are transmitted by the accidental ingestion of human faecal material. One of these is typhoid fever, which killed Willie Lincoln – he actually died from drinking water sourced from the Potomac River that was contaminated with the bacterium *Salmonella typhi*, which causes typhoid, not from the lack of a vaccine. Another is rotavirus, one of the most important causes of severe gastroenteritis in the world. Typhoid vaccines have long been in use, and vaccines against rotavirus have been developed and are being used in wealthy countries, and increasingly in poor countries too. But poor sanitation does not account for the spread of all diseases, and improved sanitation cannot prevent us from catching all infections.

We underestimate infectious diseases at our peril. In 1951, Melbourne virologist and immunologist Sir Macfarlane Burnet wrote:

> If one looks around the medical scene in North America
> or Australia, the most important current change he sees is
> the rapidly diminishing importance of infectious diseases.
> The fever hospitals are vanishing or being turned to other
> uses. With full use of the knowledge we already possess, the
> effective control of every important infectious disease, with
> the one outstanding exception of poliomyelitis, is possible.

Burnet won the Nobel Prize in 1960 for his work on immunity to infection. In 1962, his hubris persisted when he wrote: 'One can think of the middle of the twentieth century as the end of one of the most important social revolutions in history, the virtual elimination of the infectious disease as a significant factor in social life.' The end except for HIV infection, which had recently begun infecting humans at the time he wrote this (though it was not recognised as a new disease until 20 years later). The end except for pandemic influenza and mad cow disease and SARS (severe acute respiratory syndrome) and multi-resistant tuberculosis – to name just a few. Burnet was a genius, but he was fallible. Sadly, 'the virtual elimination of the infectious disease' is nowhere in sight.

To this day, vaccine-preventable infections can kill well-nourished, healthy children, or leave them permanently brain-damaged. Olivia Dahl, daughter of renowned children's author Roald Dahl, died from measles in 1962. 'Olivia, my eldest daughter, caught measles when she was seven years old,' wrote Dahl later:

> One morning, when she was well on the road to recovery, I was sitting on her bed showing her how to fashion little animals out of coloured pipe-cleaners, and when it came to her turn to make one herself, I noticed that her fingers and her mind were not working together and she couldn't do anything. 'Are you feeling all right?' I asked her. 'I feel all sleepy,' she said. In an hour she was unconscious. In twelve hours she was dead.

Olivia Dahl died from measles encephalitis, which occurs in about one in a thousand children who catch measles naturally. Tragically, measles vaccine had not been developed in 1962, but nowadays there is a highly effective and safe vaccine. For the rest of his life Roald Dahl became a staunch advocate for immunisation and particularly for measles vaccine.

Measles may be vaccine-preventable, but the vaccine has to reach children to be able to protect them. The World Health Organization (WHO) has reported that measles immunisation has prevented over 20 million child deaths since the year 2000; the annual number of measles deaths globally fell by over 80% in only 15 years from 2000 to 2015. Nevertheless, over 100,000 unimmunised children still die every year from measles in resource-poor countries.

One of the challenges with immunisation is that success can breed failure. When an effective vaccine is introduced, the targeted disease can disappear within a few years, sometimes even more quickly. Most vaccines are surprisingly safe, but no medication is totally without adverse side effects.

When examined in careful studies, the vast majority of these adverse effects cause no lasting damage. But when concerns are raised that a vaccine may be causing adverse effects, parents are likely to be worried. They are more likely to be anxious about a vaccine's safety than about a disease that they have only vaguely heard about, and from which they have never seen a child suffer.

If doctors universally believe there is no cause for concern, and tell their patients that the vaccine is safe and remind them about the severity of the disease it prevents, the public may be reassured. But when doctors are among those raising concerns, people may be confused and uncertain who to trust.

In 1974, a major controversy was ignited in the United Kingdom when a group of doctors from the prestigious Great Ormond Street Children's Hospital in London published a scientific paper in the country's leading paediatric journal suggesting that whooping cough (pertussis) vaccine might cause encephalopathy (brain disease), resulting in brain damage. Other doctors also raised concerns about the vaccine's safety.

The scientific paper described children who had neurological problems after receiving their childhood vaccines. However, it did not include a control group and did not make it clear that when one event follows another, it does not mean the first event caused the second. Subsequent research showed that children never given the whooping cough vaccine were just as likely as immunised children to develop encephalopathy, and therefore whooping cough vaccine did not cause brain damage. But the harm was done.

One of the most prominent and vocal of the doctors raising concerns was a Glasgow Professor of Public Health, Gordon Stewart. He had collaborated with Sir Alexander Fleming and had carried out trials of penicillin while working as a naval surgeon in World War II. Gordon Stewart was convinced that pertussis vaccine caused encephalopathy. He was smartly dressed, handsome, articulate and well spoken, with an endearing Scottish lilt, and the press loved him.

Stewart was no charlatan or fraud. He may have been fond of publicity, but he genuinely believed that the vaccine was dangerous, although comments like 'The risk of damage from the vaccine is now greater than the risk of damage from the disease' did nothing for public confidence.

Immunisation experts and epidemiologists tried to use the media to reassure the public that the risk was low and uncertain, but whenever the press covered the topic they presented both sides of the story 'for balance'. The anti-pertussis vaccine spokesperson always seemed to be the passionate and plausible Gordon Stewart. Whatever the reasons, rates of whooping cough immunisation in the United Kingdom fell dramatically by the late 1970s, to as low as 30% in parts of Britain.

When whooping cough immunisation had finally become available in the United Kingdom in 1950, everyone knew about the disease and the vaccine uptake was high. As a result the disease became rare. Twenty years later, parents had no memory of the horrors of having a child or a friend with whooping cough. Scared by the publicity, they perhaps understandably decided not to give their child the whooping cough vaccine. United Kingdom children in the 1970s had good diets and were well nourished, but if they were not immunised and caught whooping cough, good nutrition did not protect them. Between 1977 and 1979, over 100,000 people in the United Kingdom caught whooping cough, and at least 36 children died from it. The outbreak generated its own publicity, immunisation levels rose again and the outbreak subsided. Professor Stewart never retracted his comments, and indeed continued to publish his doubts about the vaccine's safety on an anti-immunisation website.

Another highly publicised vaccine scare was the postulated link between the measles, mumps and rubella (MMR) vaccine and autism, published by the United Kingdom gastroenterologist Andrew Wakefield in 1998, and subsequently shown to be based on fraudulent research. (I discuss that controversy in detail in Chapter 11.) By the mid 1990s, measles had all but disappeared from the United Kingdom due to high rates of immunisation; stories like the tragic death of Olivia Dahl had been almost forgotten. The autism scare resulted in a huge fall in measles immunisation rates in the United Kingdom, measles returned and children died. When the research was discredited, immunisation rates improved and measles disappeared again.

In the 1980s, Australia had a few home-grown immunisation sceptics, although the great majority of parents immunised their children. In 1996, a film-maker made a supposedly scientific documentary for the Australian Broadcasting Corporation

(ABC). She interviewed people who were both pro- and anti-immunisation in equal numbers, 'for balance'. She was pregnant with her first child, and concluded the documentary by saying that she had not yet decided whether or not to get her baby immunised. I was one of the doctors interviewed. When the documentary was shown in Australia it generated considerable debate and controversy.

Two weeks later I was in Port Moresby, the capital of Papua New Guinea, and gave a presentation to the hospital about immunisation. A number of the audience told me they recognised me from the documentary, which had been shown that week on PNG television. They were puzzled as to why anyone would make such a film. Their wards were filled with children with severe tuberculosis, newborns dying from tetanus, and babies with severe rotavirus gastroenteritis, all preventable by immunisation. On their streets were people crippled forever by poliomyelitis. But Papua New Guinea did not have the money or the public health infrastructure to deliver vaccines effectively to its population. Papua New Guineans knew vaccines could prevent the devastating diseases they saw every day, and could not understand why anyone in Australia would dream of not immunising their child.

Immunisation scepticism is very much a first-world problem.

CHAPTER 2

Smallpox, the speckled monster

The story of smallpox, one of the first diseases to be recognised by humans, is remarkable in many ways. It includes war crimes, tragedy and triumph. The introduction of smallpox devastated whole populations in Central and South America and in Australia. When it did not kill, smallpox often left a terrible legacy of facial scarring and blindness. Smallpox continued to kill millions of people every year until a half-century ago: a mere drop in the ocean of time. Within a few short years, smallpox was defeated and disappeared. The global eradication of the scourge that was smallpox is one of the greatest ever achievements of medicine, a triumph of science and public health policy.

Historical claims about smallpox are difficult to verify. Although the clinical features of the disease are reasonably characteristic, there are other infections that can mimic it, including chickenpox. Thus, although it is often claimed that Egyptian mummies had facial lesions resembling smallpox – including the mummy of Ramses V, who died in 1157 BC – it is by no means certain that Ramses really had smallpox, or that it killed him.

There are descriptions of a disease with all the characteristics of smallpox in the ancient Indian medical texts *Charaka Samhita* and *Sushruta Samhita*, which were compiled in the first century BC at the latest. The first reliable description of smallpox was in China in the fourth century AD, although there is historical evidence to suggest the disease may have been imported to China as early as the third century BC.

The horror of smallpox was that it spread through a community like wildfire, causing devastating disease. A healthy child or young adult suddenly developed severe headache, back pain, fever, nausea and vomiting, and rapidly became so weak they could hardly move. After two or three days, small red spots appeared on their face and spread rapidly to the rest of the body. The spots became enlarged, raised and blistered. Then the unfortunate victim usually died within days. People who survived were often left permanently disfigured by deep facial scars. No wonder smallpox was called 'the speckled monster'. It could also cause corneal ulceration, which rendered up to a third of all survivors totally blind.

In about 165 AD, the Roman Empire was hit by a terrifying epidemic. An army campaigning in Mesopotamia contracted a disease that it brought back to Italy. It is often called the Plague of Galen, after the Greek physician who described the epidemic. Galen treated the infected soldiers in the army camp at Aquileia in northern Italy. According to his description, the soldiers were covered with blisters that later turned into a black rash, and the blisters fell off leaving scars. Many of the soldiers had fever, bloody stools and diarrhoea, features characteristic of what we now recognise as a haemorrhagic form of smallpox. If the stools turned black, the soldier died. The epidemic killed over 6 million people; some historians assert that it was one of the more important factors leading to the decline of the Roman Empire.

Smallpox subsequently spread throughout Europe, transmitted by trade and wars, including the Crusades, and was widespread by the Middle Ages. Elizabeth I of England was imprisoned for a year by her half-sister Queen Mary, accused of supporting Protestant rebels. She succeeded Mary to the throne in 1588, aged 25. Four years later, she developed what seemed to be a bad cold. However, it rapidly progressed to a high fever, with muscle pain, malaise and headache, and she became so sick she was unable to speak.

The young queen had smallpox. Her councillors surrounded her bed, thinking she was dying. After four hours she regained consciousness and instructed her councillors, in the event of her death, to appoint a personal favourite, Lord Robert Dudley, Earl of Leicester, as Protector of the Realm (which came with a massive income of £20,000 a year). The councillors vacillated, suspecting that Dudley was a secret lover. But Bishop Quadra later wrote to the King of Spain: 'The Queen protested at the time that although she loved and had always loved Lord Robert dearly, as God was her witness, nothing improper had ever passed between them.' They must have believed her, because Elizabeth became known as both the Virgin Queen and Good Queen Bess, and reigned successfully until her death at age 69.

Elizabeth gave Dr Burcot, who tended her during her illness, a valuable land grant and a pair of golden spurs that had belonged to her grandfather Henry VII. But according to a later historian, she said that thenceforth she 'wished never to be reminded of her illness'.

Elizabeth's survival when so many around her were dying from smallpox was attributed to divine intervention. Gold medals were produced to celebrate her recovery. They showed her face as unblemished. Queen Elizabeth may have been lucky enough to avoid disfiguring facial scars. She herself said she never had wrinkles because of the smallpox. But she was not renowned for her lack of vanity and was also well aware that her reputation as a beauty carried political power. Paintings show she always wore many layers of make-up. She also showed disdain to anyone scarred by smallpox, including a suitor, the Duke of Alençon – whom she refused point-blank to marry – and one of her ladies-in-waiting, Lady Mary Sidney.

In nursing Elizabeth back to health, Lady Mary Sidney caught smallpox from her queen and was left permanently scarred. Sir Henry Sidney wrote about his wife: 'When I went to Newhaven I lefte her a full faire Ladye in myne eye at least the fayerest, and when I retorned I found her as fowle a ladie as the smale pox could make her.' Not much sympathy there.

Early in the 17th century, the first references to smallpox started to appear in English poetry. In 1616, the year William Shakespeare died, Ben Jonson published *An Epigram to the Smallpox*, in which he wrote:

Envious and foule Disease, could there not be
One beauty in an Age, and free from thee?

The English historian Lord Macaulay later wrote of this era that 'small pox was always present'. He described how smallpox disfigured both children and adults, 'turning the babe into a changeling at which the mother shuddered and making the eyes and cheeks of the betrothed maiden objects of horror to the lover'. Note the reference to the eyes as well as to facial scarring. In the 17th and 18th centuries smallpox was the leading cause of blindness in Europe.

Turlough O'Carolan (the O' is optional) was born in 1670. His father was a blacksmith from County Meath, Ireland, and worked for landed gentry, the MacDermott Roe family. The lady of the house was fond of O'Carolan and organised his education. O'Carolan was a promising young poet, but at the age of 18 he contracted smallpox, which destroyed his eyes and left him blind. The worthy Mrs MacDermott Roe sent O'Carolan to a blind school, where he was apprenticed to a harpist, Mr Cruise.

From age 21, O'Carolan became a famous itinerant musician, travelling all over Ireland on horseback with a guide, singing songs he had composed and accompanying himself on the harp. Almost all his songs were written in the Irish language. He became one of Ireland's most famous composers.

Recently I heard one of Turlough O'Carolan's compositions being played on a classical radio station. If your taste veers more towards pub music, you might well hear a Turlough O'Carolan song being performed by a band in an Irish pub.

In London in the 18th and early 19th centuries, the infant mortality rate from smallpox was 30 to 40% – one in every three babies died from smallpox before they were a year old – and in Berlin during the late 1800s a catastrophic 98% of infant smallpox victims died. In late 18th century Glasgow, half of all children died before 10 years of age, and 40% of those deaths were due to smallpox. Yet, as we have seen, adults could also die from the disease. At the end of the 18th century, the average life expectancy in France was only 32 years, largely due to smallpox.

Smallpox was unknown in the New World until it was introduced by the Spanish and Portuguese conquistadors and decimated the local population, contributing significantly to the demise of both the Aztec and Inca empires. Smallpox was introduced to the east coast of North America by early settlers, and spread rapidly through the local Native American population. The slave trade also influenced the spread of smallpox in the Americas, since many African slaves came from smallpox-affected areas.

The most severe form of smallpox, variola major, persisted in Europe and the Americas until the end of the 19th century. Variola major killed 20 to 30% of those infected, but could be even more deadly when it first spread to an island or country whose population had never been exposed to the virus and had no immunity. Such an epidemic is sometimes called a 'virgin soil' outbreak.

Two stories exemplify this island effect. In 1724, a smallpox epidemic on the island of St Kilda in Scotland's Outer Hebrides killed all but four of the men, leaving too few to bury all the islanders who had died. The second example relates to remote, sparsely populated Easter Island in the Pacific, whose Polynesian inhabitants built massive and impressive Moai stone statues. The introduction of smallpox by European sailors wiped out almost the entire population, which fell from about 3000 in 1774, when Captain Cook first landed there, to just over 100 a century later.

In 1763, during the so-called French and Indian War between British and French colonisers in North America, inhabitants of Fort Pitt (later Pittsburgh), Pennsylvania, fell ill with smallpox.

British commander Field Marshal Jeffery Amherst wrote to Colonel Henry Bouquet: 'Could it not be contrived to send the small pox among the disaffected tribes of Indians? We must on this occasion use every stratagem in our power to reduce them.' Bouquet replied: 'I will try to inoculate the Indians by means of Blankets that may fall in their hands, taking care however not to get the disease myself.'

These British Army officers excused the ethically inexcusable by declaring that the enemy were savages who did not need to be treated like human beings. Bouquet wrote to Amherst: 'that Vermine ... have forfeited ... all claim to the rights of humanity'. Amherst also wrote to Captain Simeon Ecuyer, encouraging him to send smallpox-infected blankets and handkerchiefs to the Native Americans surrounding Fort Pitt.

These letters provide incontrovertible proof that British forces planned to deliberately infect the Native Americans. While it has proved difficult to obtain robust evidence that the British definitely *did* give them contaminated blankets, most historians believe that they did, and that smallpox provided an early example of the morally repugnant practice of biological warfare.

In January 1788, the British First Fleet reached Australia, landing at Port Jackson in Sydney. The Port Jackson Aborigines were involved in resisting the European invasion. Just 15 months later, an outbreak of a disease characterised by rash and fever decimated the Aboriginal population. Based on the account of a French sailor who landed at Botany Bay soon after the start of the outbreak, Alan Moorehead wrote:

Then a disaster happened. In April 1789 black bodies were suddenly seen to be floating in the harbour and washed up

in the coves. Smallpox had struck ... by May the disease
had spread through all the harbour tribes. A few of the sick
who were too feeble to protest were brought into Sydney for
treatment but the majority, comprehending nothing of this
mysterious enormity that had struck them down, quickly
succumbed by their campfires.

Lieutenant-Colonel David Collins, a fascinating man who later
became Lieutenant Governor of New South Wales, Lieutenant
Governor of Tasmania and a deputy judge and gave his name to
St David's Church in Hobart, wrote:

> The number that it swept off by their own accounts was
> incredible. The native who at that time resided in Sydney on
> going down to the harbour to look for his former comrades
> is described by those who witnessed his emotions as suffering
> the extreme of agony. He looked anxiously into the different
> coves they visited; not a vestige on the sand was to be found
> of human foot; the excavations in the rocks were filled with
> putrid bodies of those who had fallen victims to the disorder;
> not a living person was anywhere to be met with.

Although some historians and physicians have raised the unlikely
possibility that the disease was chickenpox, the severity of the
epidemic described in historical accounts has convinced most
experts that it was smallpox. Lieutenant Watkin Tench – who
commanded five detachments of marines on the *Charlotte*, a First
Fleet vessel – wrote that doctors who examined victims found
that 'pustules similar to those occasioned by the smallpox were
thickly spread on the bodies'.

Aboriginal people had lived in Australia for more than 60,000 years, and smallpox was unknown to them. This was indeed virgin soil. The total Aboriginal population of Australia then was about 500,000. Historians estimate that the outbreak killed tens of thousands of Aboriginal people, including 90% or more of the Aboriginal population living around Port Jackson and over half of those living between the Hawkesbury River and Port Hacking. Children died from starvation when there were no adults left alive to look after them. Smallpox spread among Aboriginal populations throughout New South Wales, as far south as Jervis Bay and to the tribes on the Western Plains across the Blue Mountains, killing an unknown number.

The only case of smallpox among the immigrants was a seaman on the ship *Supply*, who died. Watkin Tench kept a journal in which he recorded that First Fleet surgeons brought with them bottles containing smallpox-infected material. In 1791 he wrote about the smallpox outbreak: 'It is true that our surgeons had brought variolous matter in bottles, but to infer that it was produced from this cause, were a supposition so wild as to be unworthy of consideration.'

Was the smallpox material intended to be used for the settlers' protection, or as another unconscionable act of early germ warfare? How smallpox spread across New South Wales – and whether the material was the cause – is contested by historians. It was only a generation since British forces wrote about infecting Native Americans with smallpox, so it is no great stretch of the imagination to believe that the Sydney outbreak was a second horrifying example of biological warfare by the British. I shudder with shame to think that my ancestors could have been capable of such an abominable act.

To this day people express concern that there are residual laboratory stocks of smallpox kept in Russia and the United States that could potentially be used in biological warfare. The rationale for keeping them is the questionable argument that they might be needed to make vaccines if smallpox re-emerged naturally, or if one of the stocks of smallpox was used for biological warfare. We know that chemical weapons are often used in modern warfare, in flagrant disregard of international law and despite international condemnation. It is frightening to contemplate the possibility that the smallpox stock might be used as a biological weapon by an unscrupulous regime, but trying to persuade the superpowers involved to destroy the smallpox stocks is about as likely to succeed as trying to persuade them to destroy their nuclear weapons.

Variolation

Such was the horror of smallpox that humans sought ways to prevent it from ancient times onwards. As we saw from the words of Thucydides in Chapter 1, it had long been recognised by physicians, scientists and indeed by historians that people who recovered from a disease were protected against it. In scientific terms, they had developed immunity.

Gradually people came to see that giving someone an *attenuated* (milder) dose of smallpox might offer some protection against the full-blown disease. This practice, known as variolation (and sometimes confusingly called inoculation) developed, probably independently, in different parts of the world, and involved a variety of techniques.

Ancient Chinese texts from the late ninth century record that particles of smallpox scabs were sometimes blown into a person's nostrils to cause an infection. This implies the Chinese recognised that smallpox is transmitted by breathing in smallpox virus carried in aerosols from pustules that have burst (an aerosol is like a fine mist of particles). Voltaire wrote that the ancient Chinese ground up smallpox scabs into a powder and took them like snuff, although he does not give the source of this information. By the 16th century, during the Ming Dynasty, variolation was a common practice in China. After about a week, the person being variolated would develop smallpox pustules and get sick, but the disease was usually milder than naturally acquired smallpox. A scar was evidence the inoculation had worked.

The Royal Society in London was founded in 1660, and would become one of the most highly esteemed scientific establishments in the world. The society was informed about variolation in China by Dr Clopton Havers in 1700. Dr Emanuele Timoni, a doctor who had studied in Padua and Oxford and practised in Constantinople, was elected as a Fellow of the Royal Society in 1703. In 1714 he described in detail in a letter to the Royal Society how variolation was carried out in Turkey.

On day 12 or 13 of the illness, the practitioner lanced the pustules of a child recovering from uncomplicated smallpox using a needle. The 'pus' was put in a clean glass bottle and closed with a tight stopper. It was quickly carried, nestled in the bosom or under the armpit to keep it warm, to the person who was to be variolated. This person's upper arm was scratched several times with a needle or lancet, inducing minor bleeding. The pus and blood were mixed and the site was covered with an object such as a half walnut shell for a few hours.

Medical opinion was divided on the benefits and risks of variolation. Smallpox was a terrible disease, but variolation was risky, and sometimes caused smallpox rather than preventing it. Naturally acquired smallpox used to kill between one in three and one in five people who caught it (20 to 30%), but would come and go in epidemics. Variolation resulted in fatal smallpox in between 1 in 50 and 1 in 200 people variolated (0.5 to 2%).

This relatively high risk posed a huge quandary. It was considerably lower than the risk of dying from smallpox infection, but the choice must have been a terrible one for parents to make. Many preferred to let nature take its course, and hope their child never caught smallpox or recovered if they did, rather than risk causing the disease themselves by having their child variolated.

It took two remarkable women to promulgate variolation successfully in the face of medical and public opposition. Lady Mary Wortley Montagu (1689–1762) was one of the great eccentric characters of her day. She came from an aristocratic background, the daughter of the Duke of Kingston, and in 1712 escaped from an intended arranged marriage by eloping with Sir Edward Wortley Montagu. She became an early feminist, a renowned and prolific letter writer and a poet, and took a keen interest in the customs and values of Muslim women.

There were two reasons why smallpox was so important to Lady Mary. In 1713, her 20-year-old brother had died from the disease, leaving two young children. Lady Mary herself had caught smallpox at age 26 and it had left her face permanently scarred (although by all accounts this did not impede her love life).

In 1716, her husband was appointed as the British ambassador to Turkey, and the couple lived in Istanbul for two years. Lady Montagu defied custom and befriended Ottoman women, visiting them in their homes, going to Turkish baths with them, and sometimes wearing Turkish costume. She learned a great deal about Turkish life and customs, and wrote letters home. These earned her some renown when they were published as *Letters from Turkey*.

In one of these letters she wrote to a friend:

> The small-pox so fatal and so general amongst us, is here
> entirely harmless by the invention of ingrafting, which is the
> term they give it. There is a set of old women who perform
> the operation. People make parties for this purpose ... the
> old woman comes with a nutshell full of the matter of the
> best sort of smallpox.

She went on to describe how the old woman opened up four or five veins 'with a large needle and puts into the vein as much matter as can lay upon the head of her needle, and after that binds up the little wound'. She concluded: 'Every year thousands undergo this operation; they take the small-pox here by way of diversion, as they take the waters in other countries.'

While in Turkey, Mary insisted that the embassy surgeon, Charles Maitland, variolate her six-year-old son, Edward, fearing he would suffer the same fate as his uncle. She did not get her daughter Mary variolated, thinking she was too young at only one month old. The Montagu family physician was the very same Dr Emanuele Timoni who had informed the Royal Society about variolation. Dr Timoni probably advised and helped Dr Maitland, although any assistance he provided has not been recorded.

When Lady Mary returned to England in 1719 she promoted variolation in her writings, but it was often dismissed as an oriental folk remedy. In 1721, when a smallpox epidemic hit London, Lady Mary asked Charles Maitland to variolate her daughter Mary, now three years old. This was the first time the procedure had been performed in England. Maitland had retired to Hertford and was nervous. He asked for three members of the Royal Society to act as witnesses before he variolated Mary in both arms. One of them, Dr James Keith, had lost all but one of his own children to smallpox, and was so impressed that he asked Maitland to immunise his surviving six-year-old son. Little Mary and Dr Keith's son both survived, and the news spread among the medical profession. The younger Mary would later marry Lord Bute, who became prime minister.

Lady Mary had influential friends, most notably Caroline, Princess of Wales, who was intelligent and interested in science. Princess Caroline spoke positively of variolation to her husband and the royal physicians, who were soon won over. Variolation had the royal seal of approval.

The royal couple were keen to publicise the technique and asked if six condemned prisoners in Newgate Prison could be offered the choice between variolation and execution. Unsurprisingly, the prisoners all chose variolation. Dr Maitland variolated three men and three women aged 19 to 36 in April 1721. Three physicians closely observed the prisoners, who all survived the treatment and were set free that September.

One of the prisoners, 19-year-old Elizabeth Harrison, was subsequently used as a human guinea-pig. She was taken to Maitland's home in Hertford, where a smallpox epidemic was raging. There she nursed a smallpox patient in the local Christ's Hospital, and lay in the same bed as a 10-year-old boy with smallpox every night for six weeks without contracting the disease. Though it's unclear whether Elizabeth had any choice in the matter, it was the strongest proof yet of the effectiveness of variolation.

The dilemma of omission (not immunising and risking the disease) versus commission (committing to accept the risk of the immunisation) was one faced by Benjamin Franklin (1706–1790), who wrote in his autobiography:

> In 1736 I lost one of my sons, a fine boy of four years old, by the smallpox taken in the common way. I long regretted bitterly and still regret that I had not given it to him by inoculation. This I mention for the sake of the parents who omit that operation, on the supposition that they should never forgive themselves if a child died under it; my example showing that the regret may be the same either way, and that, therefore, the safer should be chosen.

Benjamin Franklin was an extraordinarily talented man, renowned as a scientist, inventor and politician. He and his brothers were strong defenders of freedom of speech and published their own newspaper. In the 1720s the Franklin brothers had written in their newspaper criticising the practice of variolation for its potential to harm. It was tragically ironic, therefore, that smallpox came to Philadelphia in 1736 and killed Benjamin Franklin's beloved son Frankie.

In contrast, the great United States president John Adams had been variolated as a child, but his wife Abigail and children had not. During a smallpox epidemic in 1776, they decided that the risk of variolation was lower than the risk of catching smallpox. Abigail and her four children travelled 16 kilometres to Boston, to be inoculated by an expert, Dr Thomas Bullfinch. Purging by vomiting for a week beforehand was thought to enhance variolation, so Dr Bullfinch prescribed an emetic. Abigail's variolation was uneventful, but 11-year-old Nabby developed pustules and fevers, and her body ached terribly. John, aged nine, was fine, but the inoculation had to be repeated on six-year-old Charles and four-year-old Thomas, as in their cases the lack of a scar indicated the first inoculation hadn't worked. Charles was delirious for two days and took weeks to recover. But at the end of it all they were immune and the American public's faith in variolation grew. John Adams once famously said: 'Facts are stubborn things; and whatever may be our wishes, our inclinations, or the dictates of our passions, they cannot alter the state of facts and evidence.'

Vaccination

Variolation rapidly fell from favour when Dr Edward Jenner developed a safer and highly effective alternative called vaccination in England at the end of the 18th century. Jenner would never have developed his vaccine if it had not been for his observations of people who had been variolated, so we owe a debt to all those who practised and publicised variolation.

The names are confusing. The word 'variolation' comes from *variola*, the Latin name for the smallpox virus (*varius* means 'spotted'). *Vacca* means 'cow' in Latin, and the word 'vaccine' derives from a famous paper Jenner wrote about cowpox, a disease of cows' udders caused by the cowpox virus, which is related to but different from the much more dangerous smallpox virus. Jenner called cowpox *variolae vaccinae*. Subsequently the virus causing cowpox was identified, and was named vaccinia virus. From this name the word 'vaccination' was later coined by Louis Pasteur in honour of Jenner.

Edward Jenner was a country doctor, equivalent to a latter-day general practitioner, who worked in rural Gloucestershire. He was a careful observer and experimenter and gained the distinction of being made a Fellow of the Royal Society (FRS) in 1788. Interestingly, his FRS was awarded not for his world-changing work on vaccination, but for explaining why the young baby cuckoo has a special groove in its back. (The cuckoo's mother lays her single egg in another bird's nest; the cuckoo hatches first and uses the groove to eject the other bird's eggs.) Being an FRS allowed Jenner to present his work on cowpox to the Royal Society, which gave him scientific credibility and gave his work much more clout.

Jenner had witnessed the way smallpox could kill and maim his patients and was a keen proponent of variolation. His parents had had Jenner himself successfully variolated in 1757, aged eight, which might have influenced his enthusiasm for the practice. Jenner variolated a large number of people in his parish. Most of them developed a mild dose of smallpox, although some got severe smallpox. A third group, Jenner observed, displayed a local reaction at the site of variolation but did not develop a rash at all. From his records, Jenner was able to determine that these people had all previously had cowpox. Some were milkmaids; others had caught the disease from milkmaids. Jenner knew the folklore that milkmaids were characteristically unmarked by smallpox scars. The traditional English poem 'Where Are You Going, My Pretty Maid?' may be an illustration of this. A man courting a milkmaid asks:

'Where are you going, my pretty maid?'
'I'm going to market, sir,' she said.

'What is your fortune, my pretty maid?'
'My face is my fortune, sir,' she said.
'Then I cannot marry you, my pretty maid.'
'Nobody asked you, sir,' she said.

She has attitude, but no money.

Jenner postulated that milkmaids did not get smallpox because they had previously been infected with cowpox, which they almost universally caught from the cows they milked. The cowpox usually started on their hands, from touching the udders of infected animals, and could spread up their arms but not usually further, and they did not become ill. Some locals even reputedly infected themselves with cowpox to prevent smallpox.

Jenner did not know that both diseases were caused by viruses, nor that the viruses were related. But he did note that the appearance of the pockmarks of cowpox resembled a mild dose of smallpox, and he postulated that infection with cowpox could promote immunity against further cowpox and also against smallpox.

This was revolutionary thinking. In 1796 Jenner performed a famous experiment that would horrify a modern-day ethics committee. He lanced some cowpox pustules (fluid-filled blisters) on the hand of a milkmaid, Sarah Nelmes, sucked up the fluid and injected it into two small cuts he made in the arm of an eight-year-old boy, James Phipps. Jenner wrote of his experiment on James:

> On the seventh day he complained of uneasiness in the axilla [armpit] and on the ninth he became a little chilly, lost his appetite, and had a slight headache. During the whole of this day he was perceptibly indisposed, and spent the night with

some degree of restlessness, but on the day following he was perfectly well.

Six weeks later, Jenner inoculated James with material taken from a smallpox victim to see if James would fall ill. Fortunately the boy did not contract smallpox; the cowpox had rendered him immune. What was more, Jenner injected poor James with smallpox material more than 20 more times to make sure the immunity was long term. Edward Jenner was a thorough man, although his concern seems to have been more for the validity of his research than for the fate of wee James.

James Phipps was the son of a poor labourer who worked as Jenner's gardener, so Jenner might reasonably be accused of exploitation. However, he was generous in his gratitude: years later, Edward Jenner gave Phipps, his wife and two children a free lease on a cottage. When Edward Jenner died, James Phipps went to his funeral.

Ethics can be defined as how we believe we ought to behave. We should hesitate before using current concepts of what is and is not considered ethical to condemn historical behaviour. Was Jenner's vaccination of eight-year-old James Phipps, the child of his poverty-stricken gardener, ethical? Even if Jenner informed Mr and Mrs Phipps of the possible risks, the power imbalance is problematic. Did the Phippses fear that Mr Phipps might no longer be employed if they did not consent to the experiment? It seems unlikely that the cottage lease Jenner later gifted to the Phippses was offered at the time of the experiment, but what if Jenner offered other inducements of which we are not aware? Nowadays inducements to participate in research would raise ethical hackles, particularly if they were excessive.

A utilitarian can point to the good outcome for the Phipps family, and the even better outcome for the world: the experiment would lead to a vaccine that prevented millions of deaths. But ethicists are concerned about what we should do with 'tainted information' – data obtained through unethical research – and ponder whether such data should ever be used for ethical and beneficial results. This is not to say that Jenner's experiment was indeed unethical. However, Dr Jenner would never be able to persuade a modern research ethics committee that it was ethical to vaccinate a child before trying the vaccine on many adults first and without knowing a great deal more about the likely risks and benefits.

Jenner was not the first person to vaccinate people using cowpox. There are reliable reports of others performing similar procedures in the previous 25 years in England and Germany, including a Dorset farmer called Benjamin Jesty, who successfully gave cowpox to his wife and two children during a 1774 smallpox epidemic. Jenner was probably well aware of Jesty's experience. But even if he was not the first person to give cowpox to a child, he deserves the plaudits because he formally showed that cowpox had rendered James Phipps immune by deliberately exposing James to smallpox. Furthermore, Jenner was not satisfied with the single case of James Phipps, but tested his theory by transmitting the cowpox from person to person by inoculation.

In 1798, Jenner reported his findings on 23 subjects to a sceptical Royal Society. His paper was called *An Inquiry into the Causes and Effects of the Variolae Vaccinae, a Disease Discovered in Some of the Western Counties of England Particularly Glouchestershire* [sic], *and Known by the Name of 'Cowpox'.* The Royal Society recognised its importance, and so did the global scientific community: Jenner's paper was immediately translated into six languages and his technique of vaccination rapidly adopted throughout much of the Western world.

Nevertheless, the concept of inoculating healthy individuals with cowpox alarmed large sections of the British public. The satirist James Gillray was quick to ridicule the practice, publishing an amusing cartoon showing cow features growing out of the bodies of people being vaccinated by Jenner. Undeterred, Jenner continued to work on cowpox vaccine and publicise its use.

Catherine the Great of Russia gave the first Russian child to receive cowpox vaccine the nickname 'Vaccinov', and had the State pay for his education. Vaccines reached Newfoundland in 1800, and three years later, mass vaccination programs were started in the Spanish colonies in the Americas and the Philippines. In 1813, the United States Congress passed an Act to ensure safe smallpox vaccine supply to the American public, and in 1832 it established a vaccination program for Native Americans.

In 1803, five years after Jenner published his seminal paper, an Australian assistant surgeon, John Savage, inoculated orphans with the cowpox vaccine. New South Wales doctors needed a human supply of cowpox and there was no means of refrigeration, so they kept the cowpox vaccine alive by using a needle to transfer infectious material, which they wrongly called 'lymph', from one vaccinated person's arm to another's. A year later, Savage and another colonial surgeon, Thomas Jamison, wrote in a letter to the *Sydney Gazette* of 3 June 1804: 'It is our decided opinion, that the Cow Pox is completely established in this Colony.'

Some physicians used vaccinated children as their source of cowpox. Dr Alex Cook, a Parramatta surgeon, wrote to the *Sydney Morning Herald* in 1843:

I took a well formed scab, after falling off a child's arm
that I had vaccinated, rolled it up in a clean piece of paper
and put it into a well-corked vial. Last week I took the
same scab, (after it had been in the vial for upwards of six
months), made it into a pulp with a little warm water ...
and to my great satisfaction it produced the vaccine pustule
as well defined as if the lymph had been ever so recently
procured.

Vaccine supply was also maintained by using a truly captive
population: the women of the Female Factory in Parramatta. This
was the only convict establishment with enough unvaccinated
subjects to allow continuous propagation of cowpox.

In 1841, New South Wales Governor George Gipps heard
that Mauritius was in the throes of a virulent smallpox epidemic.
Governor Gipps offered the colonists free vaccination 'to avert
the calamities which must necessarily follow if the smallpox is
introduced into the Colony, and to keep up a constant supply
of vaccine lymph'. Doctors were told to charge a shilling for
vaccination, which would be returned if the parents brought their
child back with a scab that proved the vaccine had taken.

Gipps asked Dr JV Thompson, the Deputy Inspector General
of Hospitals, to ensure there was adequate cowpox vaccine to
protect the colony. Dr Thompson sent a letter in response. The
letter sat in the archives of the New South Wales State Records
Authority for 169 years until, on 24 November 2010, a senior
archivist, Janette Pelosi, was looking through some papers and
saw a small pink parcel pinned to a letter. The letter was titled
'Respecting Vaccine Virus' and had been written on 17 May 1841.
The accompanying package contained cowpox vaccine material

wedged between two sealed microscope slides, a common way of transporting specimens at the time.

Concerned that the virus might still be infectious, Ms Pelosi rang New South Wales Health. The package was transported breathlessly and with some publicity to the local public health unit to see if it contained viable cowpox or even smallpox. Fortunately it did not.

The historic specimen is now held at Westmead Hospital, almost next door to Cumberland Hospital, the site of the old Female Factory. The Children's Hospital at Westmead, where I work, is wedged between the two hospitals, like the cowpox specimen wedged between two microscope slides.

A year after that discovery, in 2011, the Virginia Historical Society in the United States held an intriguingly named 'Bizarre Bits' exhibition. The *Washington Post* advert noted the contents included 'an infant's smallpox scab'. This was actually a cowpox scab to be used for vaccination, enclosed in plastic and pinned to a letter written by a local Richmond man to his father in Charlottesville in 1876. An alert reader notified the US Centers for Disease Control and, to the bemusement of visitors, an emergency team arrived at the exhibition clad in gowns, masks, caps and gloves, to bag and remove the offending letter and scab. The press played up the drama. Tests showed no live virus remained.

Smallpox sceptics

There were a number of valid reasons for concern about vaccination.

Two main approaches were initially used to produce the vaccine, both of which continued to be employed until the end of the 19th century. The cowpox was either grown on calf skin, from which material was scraped and injected directly into the arms of patients, or else fluid was taken from blisters on the arm of one vaccinated patient and injected into the next patient's arm. Cow skin could carry infections, and when the vaccine was transferred from arm to arm, serious skin infections were common. The practice could also transmit other infections, including syphilis.

Some people were sceptical of the scientific basis of vaccination and had concerns about possible harms to health. Clergy often said it was against God's natural order and unchristian to use material taken from animals.

The response of the British government was to enforce the uptake of the vaccine through legislation. In 1853, Parliament passed the *Vaccination Act*, introducing compulsory smallpox vaccination for infants up to three months old. In 1867 the Act was amended to extend the age requirement to 14 years and to introduce penalties for vaccine refusal.

The legislation was highly controversial. Compulsory vaccination met with vigorous resistance, with angry opponents arguing it infringed personal liberty. The vaccination was administered under the Poor Law, also responsible for the despised public workhouses portrayed by Charles Dickens in *Oliver Twist*. Consequently, British workers associated mandatory vaccination with other manifestations of class oppression. The laws precipitated the formation of large, vociferous anti-vaccination leagues.

Advocates of smallpox vaccination who tried to use reason to persuade dissenters were doomed to frustration. In 1877, the Reverend Charles Dodgson, better known under his pen name Lewis Carroll, replied to a letter in the *Eastbourne Chronicle*, in which a Mr Hume-Rothery claimed the smallpox vaccine was giving smallpox to large numbers of people. Carroll and Hume-Rothery engaged in an increasingly heated correspondence. Carroll, 'a trifle ruffled but keeping to the point, retired after the third round'. Mr Hume-Rothery kept going until the editor gave up publishing his letters. Mr Hume-Rothery was unperturbed by being confronted with data or evidence that contradicted his cherished beliefs.

A major centre of English opposition was the Midlands industrial town of Leicester. The town's population increased sharply from the turn of the 19th century as the Industrial Revolution took hold, and drainage facilities and housing proved inadequate. Leicester developed a reputation as a hotbed of typhus and other febrile illnesses, and had one of the highest death rates among English towns.

The Leicester (later the National) Anti-Vaccination League was founded in 1869 and soon put up candidates for election to the Board of Guardians, the body that administered the *Vaccination Act*. The anti-vaccination movement championed 'the freedom for which the sons of Britain fought and bled long before our miserable local divisions rendered us a prey to the decaying laws of overbearing centralisation'.

The fates were unkind to those in Leicester who favoured immunisation. In 1872 the vaccination rate in Leicester children was over 90%. But this high rate unfortunately coincided with a local smallpox epidemic that saw 359 Leicester locals die in five years. The numbers convinced the Leicester public, wrongly, that vaccination caused smallpox. The Leicester movement grew from a handful of people to include most of the city.

The league began holding anti-vaccination rallies. At one of these, a local newspaper reported that:

An escort was formed, preceded by a banner, to escort a young mother and two men, all of whom had resolved to give themselves up to the police and undergo imprisonment in preference to having their children vaccinated. The three were attended by a numerous crowd … three hearty cheers were given for them, which were renewed with increased vigour as they entered the doors of the police cells.

In 1885, over 80,000 people marched through Leicester carrying banners, a child's coffin and an effigy of Jenner. By 1889 there had been over 6000 prosecutions in Leicester, resulting in fines in over 3000 cases and imprisonment in 64. By 1892, only 3% of Leicester children were being immunised against smallpox despite the penalties for non-compliance.

Six years later, the British Government relented and introduced exemption certificates for parents who did not wish to vaccinate their children.

In the United States, mandatory vaccination was introduced in many States between 1843 and 1855. However, William Tebb, a leading British anti-vaccinationist, visited America to give lectures against vaccination. Following his visit the Anti-Vaccination Society of America was founded in 1879. The United States approach to dissent was characteristically litigious. In several States, including California, Illinois and Wisconsin, Anti-Vaccination Society members applied to the courts to have vaccination laws repealed, without success.

In 1902, when smallpox broke out in Cambridge, Massachusetts, the local board of health mandated that all city residents be vaccinated against smallpox. One resident, Henning Jacobson, refused, arguing that the law violated his right to care for his own body. The city successfully filed criminal charges against him. Jacobson appealed to the United States Supreme Court, which in 1905 ruled that, in the event of a communicable disease, the State was legally entitled to enact compulsory laws to protect the public.

It was the first United States Supreme Court ruling ever on the power of States in relation to public health. It is surely relevant to current debates about coercion versus respect for parental autonomy.

By the early 20th century new practices were making vaccination safer. To reduce the risk of contamination, arm-to-arm transfer was banned, and vaccines were made from cowpox grown in cell cultures or in hens' eggs rather than live animals.

As the efficacy of smallpox vaccination became increasingly evident and smallpox disappeared, organised opposition to immunisation receded. The membership of anti-vaccination leagues plummeted and the leagues folded.

Smallpox eradication

Smallpox had disappeared from several Northern European countries by 1900. However, it persisted at low levels in many other wealthy countries and the incidence remained extremely high in resource-poor countries.

The first concerted effort to set up a widespread smallpox eradication program was made by the Pan American Health Organization (PAHO) in 1950. PAHO's campaign successfully eliminated smallpox from the whole of the Americas except Argentina, Brazil, Colombia and Ecuador. Despite this success, in 1958 an estimated 2 million people globally still died from the disease every year, mostly in Africa and the Indian subcontinent.

The World Health Organization (WHO) was established in 1948, and one of its earliest initiatives was to try to control smallpox. The first WHO smallpox campaign started in 1958, but had little effect due to insufficient funds. However, in 1967, the WHO introduced a new Intensified Smallpox Eradication Programme, with the ambitious aim of eliminating the disease entirely.

The team in charge of the program was known as the Smallpox Eradication Unit (SEU), based in Geneva and consisting of 812 staff from 73 countries. The overall leader was 38-year-old American Donald Ainslie Henderson (1928–2016), known all his life as 'DA'. DA was a tall, imposing man, with a stentorian voice that commanded attention. He believed in what he called a 'shoe-leather approach': actually going to the place where an epidemic was occurring, as opposed to staying put in the office. (To his wife's dismay, DA used to bring home scabs from suspected African and Asian smallpox victims and store the scabs in their fridge until he could get them tested.)

This was before computers, before mobile phones, even before fax machines. DA insisted on a 48-hour rule: the staff in the office – never more than 10 at a time – had to answer all queries, written or telephonic, within two days. Knowing the importance of feedback, DA published regular reports, an impressive 230 in all, on his team's progress.

The SEU's ambitious goal depended heavily on adequate funds, adequate vaccine supply, and a new method of surveillance to identify smallpox cases, developed by a Czech epidemiologist, Karel Raška. Initially the vaccine was provided mainly by the Soviet Union and the United States, but in the later stages of the program, over 80% of it was produced in countries where the vaccine was needed. The ability to make safe vaccines in resource-poor countries has been an important factor in the success of some later immunisation programs.

A critical advance in smallpox eradication came through a United States doctor named Bill Foege. As a teenager, Bill injured his hip and had to wear an orthopaedic body cast. Always fascinated by his uncle, a missionary in Papua New Guinea, Bill read about Albert Schweitzer's work in Africa and swore he would travel there as a doctor. It was while working on smallpox in Eastern Nigeria in 1966 that he discovered his team could stop smallpox from spreading by immunising *only* people who had been exposed to an infected person. Foege's technique of 'ring vaccination' meant that the whole population did not have to be vaccinated, saving precious resources of time and money. When one or more people in a village or town were diagnosed with smallpox, all those who might have been exposed to infection were identified and vaccinated. This was the first 'ring'. Then, a second ring of people who had possibly been exposed to the first ring was identified and vaccinated. Smallpox was thus surrounded and prevented from spreading, just as fire fighters scorch surrounding land to isolate a fire. This was an artificial form of herd immunity (see Chapter 1), and it worked a treat.

Smallpox may be an ancient disease, and one that mainly affected people in poor countries, but there are smallpox survivors alive today in Western countries who can bear witness to its ravages. In 1962, a traveller from Pakistan named Shuka Mia arrived in Cardiff, Wales. He was diagnosed with smallpox and put in isolation, and survived. A mass immunisation program was mounted throughout Wales amid fears the smallpox might spread, and 900,000 people were vaccinated.

The Rhondda Valley is some way from Cardiff, and how the disease spread there several weeks later is unknown. It also unaccountably reached nearby Bridgend. The first person to fall ill in the Rhondda Valley was 23-year-old Margaret Mansfield, who was heavily pregnant when she developed smallpox. She was admitted to the East Glamorgan Hospital, where her baby was stillborn. The family's tragedy was far from over. Margaret died soon afterwards from smallpox, and within days so did her 24-year-old sister, Patricia Pugh. Only one doctor in East Glamorgan Hospital had declined to be immunised during the mass immunisation program. He treated Margaret Mansfield, caught smallpox from her and died too.

Margaret's neighbour, 22-year-old Marion Jones, caught smallpox from Margaret, but survived. In 2002, as a 62-year-old grandmother, Marion was interviewed on BBC Television. She tried to describe the severity of her symptoms, although she had been so ill that her memory of them was hazy. What she could say was that her scars took months to heal and all her hair fell out. She also explained the devastating effect of the outbreak on the whole community. Her husband, parents and her four brothers and sisters had all caught smallpox, and all eight of them had spent over three months in hospital.

In all, 19 people died during the 1962 South Wales outbreak, most of them healthy young women.

Smallpox was eradicated from Europe by 1972, but continued to kill and scar people on the Indian subcontinent. As the disease disappeared, people there were offered a payment if they notified (reported) a case that was verified as smallpox.

The last person naturally infected with the more virulent strain of smallpox, variola major, was three-year-old Rahima

Banu from Bangladesh. In October 1975, Rahima was notified by a fellow villager, an eight-year-old girl called Bilkisunnessa, to local health authorities, who paid Bilkisunnessa for the notification.

The Bangladeshi health authorities sent a telegram to DA Henderson in America. DA sent a WHO team to the village. They confirmed the diagnosis and treated Rahima, who survived. When she was 18 years old, Rahima married a farmer and they had four children. Her fame allowed her to make money posing for photographs. Despite her fame, Rahima reported that she was stigmatised by many people, including her husband's family.

By the end of 1975, the only remaining smallpox cases, of the variola minor strain, were in the Horn of Africa, where civil war, famine and transport problems made conditions particularly difficult. An intensive program of surveillance, containment and vaccination was instituted in 1977, under the supervision of an Australian scientist, Frank Fenner (1914–2010).

The last naturally occurring case of variola minor was diagnosed in Ali Maow Maalin, a hospital cook in Somalia, on 26 October 1977. He not only made a full recovery, but also became a polio vaccinator himself. Tragically, he died in 2013, aged just 59, from malaria, which he contracted in Somalia while delivering polio vaccine.

The smallpox story was not quite over, however. In 1978 two people contracted smallpox when the virus was accidentally released from a laboratory at the University of Birmingham in England. One of them was 40-year-old medical photographer Janet Parker. Her workplace was located on the floor above the laboratory, and an inquiry found that the virus had probably spread to her darkroom from the laboratory through ducting. When Janet fell desperately ill, her parents were quarantined because they had been in contact with her. They did not catch smallpox, but while in quarantine her father had a cardiac arrest and died suddenly. The next day, Professor Henry Bedson, the scientist responsible for smallpox research at the university, went into his garden shed when his wife was distracted and killed himself by cutting his own throat. He left a suicide note: 'I am so sorry to have misplaced the trust which so many of my friends and colleagues have placed in me and my work.'

Six days after her father died, Janet Parker succumbed to smallpox. The disease had claimed its last victim.

Very few people had believed smallpox could ever be eliminated, but DA Henderson and his team had rid the world of one of its most lethal viruses within a mere 10 years. The WHO was used to a more leisurely approach to health programs, and did not know what had hit it. What had hit it was DA.

DA Henderson was one of the heroes of smallpox eradication. He played a vital role in eradicating a disease that is estimated to have killed 300 million people in the 20th century alone – an achievement of which he was deservedly immensely proud.

Another major player in smallpox eradication was Frank Fenner, a great Australian virologist who chaired the WHO Global Commission for the Certification of Smallpox Eradication, which visited and researched the evidence for smallpox eradication from all endemic (affected) countries. Frank was a modest and charming man, and would always talk to and encourage students. He was small and fastidious and always meticulously dressed. He was nothing if not comprehensive. One of his lectures went on so long he had to be carried off the podium by two men, each lifting one elbow. Frank continued giving his lecture as he left the stage. His account of the history of the eradication of smallpox commissioned by the WHO ran to over 1400 pages (something I can verify, having printed the whole document by mistake while researching this book – much to the amusement of my work colleagues).

One of Frank's greatest moments was when he was given the honour of announcing the eradication of smallpox to the World Health Assembly in 1980.

The massive global effort made to eradicate smallpox and the immensity of the achievement can hardly be over-emphasised. It is estimated that the annual cost of the smallpox campaign from 1967 to 1979 was US$23 million, and that the world saves over US$1 billion every year by no longer having to vaccinate.

But that is just the money. The saving in human suffering is immeasurable.

The eradication of smallpox is the story of Edward Jenner's careful scientific observation and his experimentation on little James Phipps, of passionate supporters like Lady Mary Montagu and equally passionate opponents, of determined and dedicated doctors like DA Henderson and Frank Fenner, of tragedies like the deaths of Janet Parker and Henry Bedson. Remarkably, thanks to immunisation, children like Rahima Banu and young adults like Ali Maow Maalin, Marion Jones and Margaret Mansfield will never again be at risk from the scourge that once was smallpox.

CHAPTER 3

The flawed genius of Louis Pasteur

On 18 October 1831, eight-year-old Louis Pasteur was terrified to hear screams coming from the outskirts of his village of Arbois, in the mountainous Jura region of eastern France. A vicious wolf had attacked the village and several villagers had suffered serious bites. If they developed rabies, they were certain to suffer a slow, terrible death that would involve frothing at the mouth and severe agitation, followed by delirium and convulsions. There was no known cure. For thousands of years those who developed rabies had died slowly and horribly, their relatives forced to sit by in helpless anguish.

Louis watched with horror as the wolf's victims, who included one of his closest friends, were taken to the blacksmith's and held down while the blacksmith cauterised their wounds. This barbaric treatment would later be shown to be totally ineffective, but it had a profound effect on Louis Pasteur. As he heard the awful screams of his neighbours when the red-hot branding iron burned their skin, and as the acrid smell of burning human flesh reached his nostrils, Louis vowed to himself he would find a way of preventing rabies.

He would honour that vow, and become one of the most important figures in the history of vaccination. Yet Louis Pasteur was a man of paradoxes and contradictions. From a humble background in rural France, he rose to become one of the greatest scientists of the 19th century, and indeed of all time. His contribution to vaccine development was invaluable, but he was not a doctor. He played a huge role in antisepsis, leading to the later development of antibiotics, but he was not a microbiologist. He was in fact a chemist, whose pioneering work on micro-organisms and vaccines reverberated through the fields of biology and medicine, and remains highly relevant to this day.

Pasteur's background would have an impact on his approach to problems later in life. His preference was always to do his research in the field, often literally. The Jura was a region of traditional crafts and trades, like tanning – his father's occupation – and winemaking, which had a chemical basis that intrigued the inquisitive Louis and which he studied and tried to improve.

Yet Pasteur was a distinctly average student. He much preferred to sit on the riverbank, fishing or drawing. He went off to school in Paris at age 16, but returned after a month because he was homesick. A year later, in 1839, he went to college in nearby Besançon and obtained a Bachelor of Arts degree in philosophy. He then obtained a Baccalauréat Scientifique (Bachelor of Science) – ironically with a poor grade in chemistry. First he was made Professor of Physics in 1848 and then Professor of Chemistry at the University of Strasbourg. Later Pasteur went to work in Paris, but he always returned to the field.

Pasteur married the university rector's daughter Marie in 1849 and they had five children. Marie was Pasteur's greatest source of support academically, and also emotionally when their two beloved daughters and one of their sons died from typhoid in childhood. Louis dictated his manuscripts to Marie in the evenings and she prepared them for publication. Much as Pasteur contributed to the world, he would have been far less effective without Marie.

Pasteur was an extraordinary scientist and thinker, and a great experimentalist in the laboratory and the field. As a chemist, he was the first person to recognise an important phenomenon we now call isomerism, which is the concept that the same molecule can exist in mirror-image forms, left- and right-handed. As a true Frenchman, he showed that fermentation worked better under anaerobic conditions (without air), and that the souring of wine that turned it to vinegar was caused by bacteria. He demonstrated that heating milk to only moderately high temperatures for a few minutes would kill any living micro-organisms and thus sterilise the milk. This sterilisation process, which was given the name pasteurisation, has played a major role in infection control and thus in vaccine manufacture.

In 1865, the Department of Agriculture sought Pasteur's help over a silkworm disease that was destroying the silk industry in France and Italy. He set up field laboratories and, over five painstaking years, established that the problem was due to infections and that the solution was to separate sick from healthy silkworms. Pasteur's work rescued the silk industry and made him even more famous.

Pasteur and immunisation

With regards to immunisation, Pasteur was especially important as the first scientist to describe attenuation, the process (mentioned in Chapter 2) whereby a sample of disease bacteria or virus is weakened by heat, chemical treatment or other processes, and can then be used to inoculate people against the full-strength form of the disease. This discovery came from a serendipitous observation – although as Pasteur once said, with no trace of false modesty: 'In the fields of observation, chance favours only the prepared mind.'

While working on chicken cholera, a disease that could spread through a farmyard and wipe out an entire flock in three days, Pasteur was able to identify and grow the cholera bacillus (a rod-shaped bacterium). If he injected chickens with the bacillus they died within 48 hours.

When Pasteur left Paris to escape the heat in the summer of 1879, he left his cultures on the laboratory shelf. After he returned and inoculated chickens with the stored bacilli, the chickens remained healthy. He and his team grew new cultures of the bacillus and tested them on new birds, as well as on those that had survived inoculation with the cultures from the shelf. The new birds all died, but the birds previously inoculated again remained healthy. Repeatedly growing the cultures had weakened, or attenuated, the bacilli, Pasteur realised. This in turn protected the inoculated birds against the virulent bacillus strain.

Pasteur also recognised that his observations resembled those made some 80 years previously by Edward Jenner, and indeed (as mentioned earlier) it was Pasteur who coined the term 'vaccination' in honour of Jenner. Pasteur's finding has been used to make attenuated viral vaccines like those currently used against measles, mumps, rubella and chickenpox.

Pasteur next set his mind to the problem of anthrax, a disease decimating the sheep and cattle industries. The German physician–microbiologist Robert Koch, a rival and fierce critic of Pasteur, had isolated the anthrax bacillus, but it was Pasteur who proved that the organism was the cause of the disease.

Typically making observations while walking in the country, Pasteur noticed that one corner of a field where sheep were grazing was a different colour from the rest. When he made inquiries, the farmer tending the pasture told him he had buried some sheep that had died from anthrax in that corner.

Pasteur deduced that worms feeding on the carcasses of the infected sheep were bringing anthrax spores to the surface, and that sheep grazing on the contaminated soil were becoming infected. But stopping the sheep from feeding on contaminated soil would not be enough to prevent disease transmission, so Pasteur put his energy into developing a vaccine, attenuating the anthrax bacillus by oxidising and ageing it.

The vaccine was promising in the laboratory, but a well-known veterinarian called Hippolyte Rossignol was sceptical and challenged Pasteur to test his vaccine in a public trial. Pasteur agreed.

The venue for the trial was a farm called Pouilly-le-Fort south of Paris, the year 1882. The trial would involve 50 sheep; Pasteur would vaccinate half, and the other half, the control group, would remain unvaccinated. All the sheep would then receive a large, usually lethal dose of anthrax. The challenge was that all the control sheep had to die and all the inoculated sheep survive.

The press had a field day (dad joke). Not only the French papers but also the London *Times* published daily bulletins. Excited crowds created a carnival atmosphere.

They were not disappointed. Within two days, all 25 control sheep were dead and all 25 inoculated sheep still alive. One can imagine the headlines: 'Pasteur Prevails in the Pasture'! This triumph did wonders for Pasteur's reputation, but nothing for his humility.

Over the next 10 years, 3.5 million sheep and 500,000 cattle were vaccinated against anthrax, of which more than 99% survived. Mass immunisation was born.

Pasteur and Australia

In 1888 Pasteur sent his assistant, Dr Adrien Loir, on a steamer from Paris to Sydney with cultures of chicken cholera. Loir was Madame Pasteur's nephew (the word 'nepotism' derives from the popes' practice of favouring their illegitimate sons, who were called their nephews, or *nipoti* in Italian). Loir and Pasteur had made a bid for a £25,000 prize offered by the New South Wales Government's Intercolonial Rabbit Commission for anyone who could demonstrate a plausible way to eliminate rabbits.

In 1859, an English settler called Thomas Austin had had 24 rabbits sent out from the United Kingdom and released them on his property, Barwon Park in Victoria, so he could hunt them for 'sport'. By the time the rabbit commission was set up in 1887 – less than 40 years later – they had bred like, well, rabbits, numbering more than a billion and occupying over two-thirds of Australia.

Pasteur and Loir's rabbit proposal involved infecting rabbits with food laced with chicken cholera. The New South Wales

Government set up a laboratory on Rodd Island in Iron Cove, Sydney, and it was in this laboratory that Loir made the chicken cholera virus.

In a preliminary experiment, Loir also offered the food to native birds and poultry. Rabbits that ate the food died, but not rabbits that avoided it, whereas every test bird died. The rabbit commission refused to award Pasteur the prize. It is just as well his proposal was rejected: one man-made ecological disaster was already one too many.

Soon after Loir's arrival in Australia, Arthur Devlin, a grazier, contacted the Pasteur Mission to report that his properties were being affected by a sheep disease referred to locally as 'Cumberland disease'. Realising that the disease was anthrax, Loir carried out a field trial at Junee Junction in country New South Wales, similar to Pasteur's Pouilly-le-Fort trial. A local board was appointed; its chairman, in a wonderful case of nominative determinism, was a sheep grazier called John de Villiers Lamb.

The vaccine trial was carried out on 39 sheep and six cows. Vaccinated sheep were shorn for identification. Every vaccinated sheep and cow survived. All the unvaccinated sheep and one unvaccinated cow died. Pasteur was asked to supply anthrax vaccine for the whole colony. He said he would arrange it, but when his bid for rabbit eradication was rejected he had a fit of pique and changed his mind. Eventually he was persuaded by a sizeable financial inducement to set up a laboratory in Australia to manufacture anthrax vaccine. This finally led to the manufacture of anthrax vaccine at a new establishment, the McGarvie Smith Institute.

(Loir was not averse to more scandalous experimentation. In 1891, the most famous and controversial personality of the day,

French actor Sarah Bernhardt, arrived in Australia for a tour. She brought two dogs and, just as would happen to Johnny Depp and Amber Heard with their two dogs in 2017, fell foul of Australian quarantine regulations. Loir, a smitten fan, persuaded health authorities to quarantine Sarah Bernhardt's dogs on Rodd Island. Sarah Bernhardt, who had a penchant for younger men, missed her acting engagements in Brisbane while the pair had a short, passionate affair.)

Pasteur and rabies

In 1868, aged just 46, Louis Pasteur suffered a stroke, which left him with speech impairment and permanently paralysed down one side. His faithful wife, Marie, nursed him back to physical and psychological strength. Quite extraordinarily, he would carry out all his future work while still paralysed.

Pasteur had never forgotten the tragic deaths he had witnessed as an eight-year-old in Arbois, after the wolf attacked the village. Forty-odd years later, rabies infection was still a terrible scourge. In London, for example, 29 people died of rabies in early 1877, stimulating the passing of a 'Rabies Order' that permitted police officers to dispose of stray dogs by any means possible in order to combat 'rabies of the streets'.

Pasteur's next great project – and perhaps the crowning achievement of his career – would be to develop a rabies vaccine. He was assisted in this work by a young colleague named Emile Roux, a medical doctor as well as a practising physician, bacteriologist and immunologist.

Pasteur and Roux showed that the organism responsible for rabies could be found in the spinal cord and brain of affected animals. Seeking to create a vaccine, the two men experimented with strips of spinal cord from rabid rabbits and made a fascinating discovery, as Pasteur reported to the French Academy of Sciences in 1885:

> The spinal cords of these animals are rabid throughout their length with a constancy in their virulence. If, taking the greatest possible care to maintain purity, one removes from these cords sections a few centimetres in length, and then suspends them in dry air, virulence slowly reduces until it finally disappears.

The longer the cord was dried, the less potent it was in causing rabies when injected into test animals. To work out the ideal level of attenuation, Pasteur and Roux injected dogs with cord extracts of gradually increasing potency; then they created a vaccine.

Rabies vaccine is different from most vaccines, which are usually given well before exposure to the organism in order to protect against it. Because the incubation period of rabies is weeks or even months, it is possible to protect someone bitten by a rabid animal by giving vaccine even quite a long time after the exposure. In July 1885, Pasteur was visited by three people who had travelled over 500km from Alsace to Paris, Theodore Vone, nine-year-old Joseph Meister and Joseph's mother. Monsieur Vone's dog had developed rabies and had attacked poor Joseph, who had been bitten 14 times, so severely he could hardly walk.

Pasteur was not a medical doctor but was persuaded to try his rabies vaccine on Joseph. Pasteur later wrote: 'As the death of this child seemed inevitable, I decided, not without deep and severe unease, as one can well imagine, to try on Joseph Meister the procedure which had worked consistently in dogs.'

Emile Roux gave Joseph a dose of rabies vaccine – the first ever dose given to a human. Joseph was given 12 more injections of vaccine over the following 10 days, and survived.

A few months later, in October 1885, Pasteur received a letter from the Mayor of Villers-Farlay, a small town near Arbois. The mayor asked if Pasteur could help a brave 15-year-old shepherd, Jean-Baptiste Jupille, who had been bitten while saving the lives of six younger shepherds being attacked by a rabid dog. Pasteur agreed, and Jean-Baptiste took the next train to Paris. Emile Roux immunised him daily with injections of the rabies vaccine.

On the sixth day of treatment, Pasteur presented a famous paper to the French Academy of Sciences, in which he described young Jean-Baptiste's courage and the basis for giving him the new rabies vaccine:

> The Academy perhaps cannot hear without emotion the account of the courageous act and great spirit of the young man whom I have begun to treat last Tuesday. He is a 15-year-old villager called Jean-Baptiste Jupille from Villers-Farlay (Jura) who, seeing a large fierce dog acting suspiciously and threatening a group of six of his little friends, all much younger than him, threw himself, armed only with his whip, in front of the animal. The dog seized Jupille by the left hand. Jupille then threw the dog to the ground, held him down, opened his jaws with his right hand in order to free his left hand, not without receiving many new bites, then with the cord of his whip, muzzled him and striking him with his shoes, killed him.

> After innumerable experiments, I have finally found a
> method that has already proved successful so consistently in
> so many dogs that I feel confident of its general applicability
> to all animals and to man himself.

After hearing this account, one member asked the academy to award Pasteur the national prize for virtue, which seems a bit excessive, even for the French. Although this was not granted, Pasteur's efforts did not go unrewarded. The academy publicised the news of Pasteur and Roux's vaccine and it spread rapidly around the world. It is indicative of Pasteur's international standing and his ego that he took the lion's share of the credit, even though Roux made enormous contributions to the research. Pasteur and Roux's rabies vaccine was just the second human vaccine in the world, after Jenner's smallpox vaccine.

People bitten by rabid animals travelled to Paris from far and wide asking to be given the vaccine, including a group of Russian peasants who had been severely mauled by a rabid wolf. Their leader knew a single French word: 'Pasteur'. Pasteur organised for them to receive his vaccine and all but three survived. The Russian Tsar was so impressed that he awarded Pasteur the Diamond Cross of St Anne, and donated the small fortune of 100,000 francs to aid Pasteur's research.

Pasteur was now revered in France and worldwide. When he died in 1895, aged 72, his body lay in state on an elaborate bier before being carried along Paris boulevards lined with thousands of grieving citizens. His funeral was attended by the President of France, princes from Greece and Russia, and Lord Joseph Lister, the great pioneer of sterile surgery, whose own work owed so much to Pasteur.

Emile Roux's loyalty did not go unrewarded, because despite suffering from chronic lung disease, he co-founded the Pasteur Institute in 1887, worked there for nearly 50 years and became director, after his mentor Emile Duclaux, who himself had succeeded Pasteur. Roux would achieve fame in his own right for his work on the often fatal disease diphtheria (as we shall see in Chapter 6).

There was a tragic end, however, to the story of Joseph Meister, the first person injected with the rabies vaccine. Meister spent most of his life working as a caretaker at the Pasteur Institute before committing suicide there in 1940, aged 64. One version of the story concerning his suicide is that German troops ordered him to open Pasteur's tomb. Joseph refused and committed suicide instead. A less romantic and better documented version has it that Meister was racked with guilt at having sent his family away from Paris, as he was convinced they had been killed. In a sad piece of irony, they returned unharmed the same day he took his own life.

Only human

A thorough analysis of Louis Pasteur's secret notebooks has shown that the great scientist was sometimes dishonest about the details of his experiments, secretly made use of other people's work and failed to acknowledge significant contributions from colleagues like Roux. As an example of his dishonesty, Pasteur and Roux wrote that they had been completely successful in protecting 50 dogs against rabies, but Pasteur's own records later showed he had tested only 11.

While it is disappointing to hear that a great scientist was not all he pretended to be, Pasteur was by no means the first such case. It is interesting that he was apparently so convinced his theories were correct he was prepared to falsify his data. He presumably felt that inflating numbers was not cheating but exaggeration. Can someone who behaved as unethically as Pasteur sometimes did be considered a truly great scientist? Or are we just being naïve in creating heroes to worship without making due allowance for human frailty?

However flawed he was, there is no doubting the immense contribution Louis Pasteur has made to human health, the deaths he has prevented and the misery he has averted. His experimental rigour is honoured in the French government-funded Pasteur Institute, a model of scientific and medical research that has been emulated in many European countries, where these institutions are the major centres of scientific research (unlike in North America, where universities have come to dominate research).

Pasteur has been called the Father of Immunology, and one of his greatest legacies is the crucial role he played in the development of vaccines and the process of immunisation.

CHAPTER 4

The end of polio

It was 1921. Franklin Delano Roosevelt – FDR, as he was fondly known – was 39 years old and a highly promising young politician. His stocks in the Democratic Party were rising and he had the whole world before him. However, on the fateful day of 10 August all that would change.

FDR was holidaying with his wife, Eleanor, and their five young children on Campobello Island in Maine when they went sailing in the family yacht. On their return to the island, FDR went for a swim in a pond with the children and raced the boys home, 3 kilometres away.

That evening he had fever and chills and his lower back was very sore. He felt nauseous and did not eat supper, but went straight to bed.

Next morning one of his legs was weak. By evening he was unable to move it and the other leg was also weak. He was racked by fevers and chills. His legs, when not numb, were excruciatingly painful, and so was his back. He was unable to urinate and had to be catheterised. He was also severely constipated, needing enemas. His arms and shoulders grew weak, he became paralysed from the chest down, and he had difficulty breathing.

At first the doctors prescribed physiotherapy, which caused Roosevelt agonising pain. Then he was transferred to New York, where doctors diagnosed polio. He improved slowly, and spent weeks trying to walk, but was unable to win that battle and never walked again.

FDR was adamant that his disability would not stop his political career. Undaunted, he was determined to be seen as a normal man who just happened to be in a wheelchair. His upper body strength and physique became legendary. He went fishing, fought a shark that weighed over 100 kilograms for two hours solo and landed it successfully.

His political advisers thought his physical infirmity would be interpreted as weakness and wanted to distance him from his polio. They made sure photographs only showed him from the waist up.

His political career thrived. His courageous attitude to his illness won rather than lost him votes. He was a charming and engaging man. In 1929 he became Governor of New York, and in 1932 he won a landslide victory to become the first ever disabled President of the United States.

FDR had many claims to fame, but one of his most lauded achievements was that he introduced the 'New Deal' policy that helped the United States out of the dreadful 1930s economic collapse. How telling that a disabled president should find a solution to the Depression.

FDR devoted much energy to fighting polio. In 1927 he launched a hospital and research facility in Georgia dedicated to polio research, called the Warm Springs Foundation. In 1938, two years after being re-elected by an even bigger margin, he founded a not-for-profit organisation he called the National Foundation for Infantile Paralysis, in order to raise funds to combat polio.

He invited wealthy celebrities to events on his birthday each year. At one of these fundraisers, vaudeville comedian Eddie Cantor, famous for his blackface minstrel songs, suggested jokingly that the public should send dimes (10-cent pieces) directly to the president. The inspiration may have been 'Brother Can You Spare a Dime?' (or 'Buddy Can You Spare a Dime?'), a famous song of the Depression.

The public, for whom polio was visible daily in the bodies of their friends, their family and their president, took Eddie Cantor literally. The White House was swamped with bags of mail full of dimes – nearly 3 million in total – and could barely cope. The name of the National Foundation for Infantile Paralysis was changed to the March of Dimes, a play on the name of a popular radio series called *The March of Time*.

An early March of Dimes fundraising effort was selling badges for a dime. Every Christmas, booths were set up with slots where children could insert a dime to buy a badge.

This extraordinary appeal to the masses has to date generated over 7 billion dimes, and the March of Dimes has donated US$500 million towards combating polio. It was one of the earliest and remains one of the most impressive examples of 'crowd-funding'.

In fact, FDR's diagnosis of polio was never confirmed, and some modern physicians have suggested his illness was more likely to have been Guillain-Barré syndrome, a nervous disease of unknown cause. The appropriate tests, such as a lumbar puncture, were not done, so the true diagnosis is speculative. The symmetrical nature of the paralysis and the way it ascended from FDR's legs to involve his chest and face are more typical of Guillain-Barré syndrome, whereas the fevers and chills and permanent paralysis favour polio.

Regardless of the true diagnosis, FDR's illness made polio famous, and he himself made a huge contribution towards eradicating the disease.

Bert Flugelman

Herbert (Bert) Flugelman was born in Austria in 1923 and fled to Australia in 1938 to avoid the coming world war. He became a budding sculptor and moved to England in 1951. A year later, aged 29, he was suddenly struck with polio, mostly affecting the muscles of his left leg and his trunk. Doctors in a London hospital told Bert he would never walk again.

Refusing to accept this, Bert discharged himself from hospital. He had a bed erected on the roof of his London house and, with the help of friends, gradually got back on his feet. He would thenceforth always have a tilt and walk with a limp, but he steadfastly refused to let polio impair his art, which, on the contrary, flourished. Bert's courageous approach is reminiscent of Australian author Alan Marshall who, in his wonderful book, *I Can Jump Puddles*, describes the horror of realising he could not use his legs after contracting polio at age six and his courageous battle to live as normal a life as possible thereafter.

Over the next three years Bert exhibited at the Piccadilly Gallery in London and the Barone Gallery in New York. He returned to Australia in 1955 and fashioned a career as an academic and a major sculptor. His magnificent work *Cones* has been exhibited in the Sculpture Garden at the National Gallery of Australia in Canberra since 1982. Bert exhibited on several occasions at Sculpture by the Sea in Bondi, New South Wales; a photo of one of his pieces, *Tetrus*, is used to advertise the event each year.

In 1977 Bert was commissioned to make a sculpture to adorn a new pedestrian precinct in Adelaide, Rundle Mall. Bert produced two superimposed silver balls. His favoured title for the work was *On Further Reflection*, but the authorities preferred the simple *Spheres*. On the day the sculpture was unveiled, the Adelaide *Advertiser* used the headline 'Bert's Balls in the Mall', a story Bert would often tell with a wicked grin. The sculpture has become an Adelaide icon, and has forever since been known as Bert's Balls or The Mall's Balls. The image appears on postcards, key-rings and posters, sometimes using the phrase 'Adelaide's Got Balls'.

For years Bert and his partner Rosie lived in splendid isolation in a small hillside community in New South Wales called Jamberoo, only accessible by four-wheel drive, where lyrebirds would scamper across the road. He had few neighbours, but one was a close friend and fellow artist, Guy Warren, a painter. Bert had achieved his fame as a sculptor, but had painted in his youth. One evening over dinner, when a bottle or two of wine had been consumed, Bert bet Guy that he could paint as well as Guy could. Guy issued a challenge that they would each paint the other and submit their portraits to the highly prestigious Archibald Prize for portraiture at the Art Gallery of New South Wales. Bert's painting did not make the cut, but Guy's portrait of Bert won the 1985 Archibald Prize. Bert's stance shows the characteristic body tilt that is a legacy of polio, with the muscles wasted more on one side of the body than the other. Guy depicts Bert with wings, inspired by the hang-gliders who would leap off Jamberoo Mountain, but with a possible nod to Icarus. Guy called his portrait *Flugelman with Wingman*.

Only later did Bert tell Guy that the name had special resonance because Flugelman means 'flying man' in German.

All about polio

Polio is almost as ancient as smallpox. People with limbs withered by the disease are depicted on Egyptian stone carvings called steles dated to 3500 years ago.

Polio – or poliomyelitis, to give its full scientific name (from the Greek meaning 'inflammation of the grey matter of the spinal cord') – has often been called infantile paralysis, although FDR's and Bert's stories show it could also hit adults.

The list of famous people who had polio as children and went on to lead highly productive lives is a long one. It includes actors Alan Alda, Mia Farrow and Donald Sutherland; musicians Neil Young, Ian Dury, Joni Mitchell and Pinchas Zukerman; artist Frida Kahlo; authors Sir Walter Scott and Arthur C Clarke; politicians Kim Beazley and Paul Martin; and sporting personalities Jack Nicklaus and Wilma Rudolph. But these stories of famous people who have heroically conquered adversity hide the extent of the human misery caused by a truly dreadful disease. Polio is the 'cripple', legs crumpled underneath him, crawling across courtyards and up church steps in Mexico. Polio is the deformed beggar with a withered, stick-thin leg and contorted spine begging in the streets of India or Africa, China or Vietnam. Polio is the child hobbling along on crutches. Polio is babies, children and young adults in iron lungs because they cannot breathe for themselves.

Those are the survivors. In a chapter entitled 'Little White Coffins' in his book *The Cutter Incident*, Paul Offit quotes a New York social worker who said of a young mother in 1916: 'There were three little hearses before the door; all her children had been swept away.' In his novel *Nemesis*, American Pulitzer Prize–winning author Philip Roth recounts a polio outbreak in Newark in 1944. Roth describes the sheer terror polio creates in the frightened, bewildered community. There is a desperate dearth of information. Parents are powerless as the disease spreads rapidly and seemingly at random, sentencing child after child to die or be crippled.

Polio is an infectious disease caused by the poliovirus, which enters the body through the intestinal tract (gut). It is caught by inadvertently swallowing food or water infected with faecal matter from an infected person. The virus can stay in the faeces for some weeks, during which time it can be transmitted to other people. While polio is thought of today as a disease of poverty, in the past it affected rich and poor alike, due to the lack of safe water and sanitation.

Most infected people stay asymptomatic (have no symptoms) and recover without any long-term ill effects. But a sizeable number develop an influenza-like illness with fever, sore throat, headache, vomiting, fatigue and limb pain. A few will experience neck stiffness due to meningitis. One in 200 of those infected develops flaccid paralysis (floppy weakness) of their muscles. The paralysis usually affects several muscles and is characteristically asymmetric, affecting one side of the body more than the other, as shown by what happened to Bert Flugelman. The muscles often become wasted through lack of use.

Polio most commonly affects one or both legs, and can result in skinny, deformed legs. At its worst the legs will become twisted up under the poor victim, who has to drag himself or herself along on his or her hands. The arms can also be affected, but this is less common. The trunk is the next most common site, and this can lead to a bend in the spine called a scoliosis, resulting in a tilted body.

If the breathing muscles are involved the patient might be unable to breathe adequately, which is why some people used to be kept alive in an artificial respiration machine called an iron lung. (Most were able to breathe on their own after a few weeks, but an unfortunate few spent the rest of their lives in the machines.) Occasionally the swallowing nerves are affected, causing what is called a bulbar palsy. Poliovirus damages the motor nerves (the nerves that make the muscles work), though the sensory nerves remain intact. Patients often have excruciating muscle spasms: imagine having cramp that persists for weeks.

We do not know why some people develop paralysis and others remain well, although it has been shown that paralysis tends to occur where there has been recent trauma, for example in a leg that has received an injury or an intramuscular injection. It has even been known to occur in the muscles used for swallowing if the victim catches polio just after a tonsillectomy. I looked after one poor boy affected in this way, and he had to be fed by a tube through his nose because he could not swallow properly.

Many people who develop paralytic poliomyelitis recover at least some of their muscle function, but for an unfortunate few the paralysis is lifelong. To add insult to injury, some polio sufferers have a recurrence of weakness late in life, a condition called post-polio syndrome.

When I was a schoolboy in rural Hertfordshire in England, there was a home neaby for people handicapped by polio. A sign on the road warned drivers: 'CRIPPLES CROSSING'. One day a motorist stopped and asked for directions, because he could not find a place called Cripples Crossing on his map. The staff laughed when they heard about it, but polio is no laughing matter for those permanently disabled by it.

Sister Kenny

As well as many victims, some of whom showed remarkable heroism, polio produced heroes who fought to overcome the ravages of the disease. Elizabeth Kenny (1880–1952), the daughter of a poor Irish farmer and his Australian wife, was born in Warialda, New South Wales. Her parents called her Lisa. The family later moved to a small town called Nobby near Toowoomba in Queensland, where her mother home-schooled her.

At the age of 17, Lisa broke her arm while horse-riding. During her long convalescence in Toowoomba, her orthopaedic surgeon, Aeneas McDonnell, lent her his textbooks. She was intrigued by the drawings of the bones and muscles and how they worked, and started to teach herself anatomy. She asked Dr McDonnell if she could borrow a skeleton to see how the bones moved, but he told her this was not allowed – skeletons were strictly reserved for medical students. Undaunted, she made her own model skeleton from ropes and pulleys.

Later she volunteered at a small maternity hospital in country New South Wales and learned nursing on the job. By the age of 30 she had set up her own practice at the family home in Nobby. She was a true 'bush nurse'. She never formally qualified, but wore a nurse's uniform she'd had made. She did not charge any money, and would ride on horseback to see any patients who requested her help.

In 1911 she was asked to see a young girl on a farm and found the girl was paralysed. She had never seen anything like it, and contacted Dr McDonnell for his opinion. He replied: 'It sounds like infantile paralysis. There's no known treatment, so do the best you can.'

Elizabeth used hot packs to relieve the girl's muscle spasms and moved her limbs to mobilise her. To everyone's relief, the girl recovered. When twenty more children in the district developed polio, Elizabeth treated six of them, who all improved.

Stimulated by her success, she opened a cottage hospital in the nearby town of Clifton. However, soon afterwards war broke out. She asked Dr McDonnell to write a letter vouching for her nursing prowess and in 1915 was appointed as a staff nurse in the Australian Army Nursing Service. Elizabeth worked on troopships, tending to wounded soldiers who were being transported back to Australia. In 1917 she was promoted to first lieutenant in the nursing service, which carried with it the title of sister.

After the war, she went back to Nobby and resumed her home nursing career. She proudly called herself Sister Kenny for the rest of her remarkable life.

Sister Kenny's inventiveness was exemplified in 1927 when she designed and patented a special ambulance stretcher, the Sylvia Stretcher, to try to reduce shock in patients requiring transport. This innovation was prompted by an accident on a neighbour's property. Seven-year-old Sylvia Kuhn sustained horrific injuries when she was standing behind her father on a plough and her dress caught in the machinery. Sister Kenny took the door off a room in the farmhouse and strapped Sylvia to it to stabilise her for transport by truck to hospital. Sister Kenny decided the existing stretchers were not suitable for carrying a badly injured and shocked patient, and within weeks she had designed her own. She patented it in Australia, New Zealand, the United Kingdom, France, Canada, India and South Africa. The prestigious London-based Institute of Patentees and Inventors awarded Sister Kenny their Gold Medal. The regular royalties from the stretcher plus her war pension were often her sole source of income while she was working on the treatment of polio.

Sister Kenny moved to Townsville, and in 1934 she leased a room in the Queen's Hotel on the seafront and set up a clinic treating patients recovering from polio paralysis and cerebral palsy. It was the first nurse-led research establishment in Australia.

The prevailing medical opinion was that patients should be immobilised and should wear splints, callipers and braces to try to correct deformities. Sister Kenny thought this was nonsense. She felt that immobilising the muscles would only make things worse. She used hot baths and hot cloths to relax patients' muscles, moved their affected limbs passively and persuaded the patients to move their own muscles actively. (This was what Bert Flugelman was later to do for himself.) We now know that the muscle wasting and contractures (permanently bent joints) of polio are exacerbated by lack of use, so Sister Kenny was absolutely correct.

The Queensland Government sponsored a meeting in Brisbane for Sister Kenny to demonstrate her methods to doctors, but she was ridiculed. To be fair to the doctors, Sister Kenny talked about 'incoordination', 'mental alienation' and 'spasm' – terms of her own invention – as the causes of paralysis, which made the doctors doubt her expertise. She even claimed that strength was transferred from her massaging fingers into the patient's muscles, which was way too mystical for your average Queensland doctor. On the other hand, when did white male doctors ever listen to a woman, let alone one who was not even qualified?

Totally unfazed, Sister Kenny responded vehemently to their criticism, using her impressive results as her argument. She was supported by the parents of children whom she had treated, and within two years the Queensland Government had set up polio treatment clinics using her techniques in Townsville and Brisbane. The Brisbane clinic attracted polio victims from other states and even from overseas. Soon more 'Kenny clinics', as they were by then known, opened in Queensland and other States.

In 1937, Elizabeth Kenny published a book, *Infantile Paralysis and Cerebral Diplegia*. She was invited to England to demonstrate her 'Kenny method'; grateful parents paid her fare. The English doctors were just as shocked as their Queensland counterparts at her recommendations to mobilise patients and stop using splints.

When she returned to Australia she found that a royal commission had accepted the opinion of Queensland doctors who condemned the Kenny method. Yet the Superintendent of Brisbane General Hospital, ignoring both the doctors and the royal commission, gave Sister Kenny her own ward so that she could continue to treat patients.

In 1940, the Queensland Government, more impressed by her results than the report, paid Sister Kenny's fare to the United States to visit the Mayo Clinic in Rochester, Minnesota. Six Brisbane doctors were sufficiently impressed by Sister Kenny to write letters of recommendation, which she took with her.

The United States doctors were also dubious about the language Sister Kenny used to describe how polio caused disability, but three orthopaedic surgeons arranged for her to treat some patients in Minneapolis General Hospital and her excellent results soon convinced the doubters. The patients improved and went home more quickly than those not treated using the Kenny method.

The United States became enamoured of this tall, imposing Australian woman with white hair, who would speak gently to a child with polio one minute and berate a doctor ferociously the next. In Chicago she met Dr Morris Fishbein, editor of the *Journal of the American Medical Association*, who said, 'She came in wearing that hat that made her look like Admiral Nelson. She *looked* like a screwball.' In 1942 the Sister Kenny Institute was opened in Minneapolis, the first of a number of Kenny clinics in the United States. A year later Sister Kenny published her autobiography *And They Shall Walk*. The story of her remarkable contribution was told in a feature film made in 1946 called *Sister Kenny*, in which she was played by Rosalind Russell. When Kenny attended the premiere in New York, a crowd of 20,000 fans broke down the barriers in their efforts to get close to her.

By 1947, the Kenny method had become so popular in the United States that 10,000 polio splints were sold for scrap metal. The Kenny method was also widely adopted in Central and South America, particularly Costa Rica and Argentina.

Eleanor Roosevelt was the most admired woman in the United States for 20 years according to Gallup polls. In 1952, however, she was displaced by Sister Elizabeth Kenny. The people of America even raised funds to buy her a prayer book that had belonged to Florence Nightingale.

Although she was revered in the United States, Kenny remained a controversial figure in Australia, where few people have ever heard of her. She never married, but in 1926 she answered an advertisement in the newspaper to adopt seven-year-old Mary Stewart (who came from a destitute Brisbane family), thus becoming the first ever single Australian woman permitted to adopt a child.

Kenny took Mary with her to the United States. Mary was devoted to her adoptive mother and said she saved her life. Mary herself became a Kenny nurse. Sister Kenny developed Parkinson's disease, retired to Toowoomba in 1951 and died in 1952.

In her heyday, she must have been a nightmare for the doctors she confronted, but she made more of a difference in the treatment of polio than all of them put together – so much so that the Kenny method became the foundation of modern physiotherapy.

The first vaccines against polio

Although much progress was made by Sister Kenny and others in treating polio victims, prevention was always going to be preferable, and a vaccine was sorely needed.

The story of polio vaccines is the story of two competing approaches, and of a great rivalry between two great men.

The first possible approach to making a polio vaccine was to produce attenuated poliovirus (like Pasteur's attenuated rabies virus) that could be given orally. The alternative was to kill the virus, which would make a safer vaccine that would be less likely to cause polio accidentally. But then the vaccine would need to be injected, as a killed vaccine cannot be absorbed from the gut.

Albert Sabin moved to New Jersey in the United States from Poland with his family in 1920, aged 15, to escape the vicious pogroms being waged against the Jewish community. He was already engaged in polio research when Jonas Salk was finishing high school. Eight years younger, Salk was also Jewish, the eldest son of a Russian immigrant family which had likewise fled pogroms. His uneducated parents had worked tirelessly to send him to one of the finest high schools in New York.

While Salk was still training in virology research, the two men met at a polio conference in 1948. At one point, Salk asked Sabin whether an alternative method for mapping strains of polio virus could be found.

Sabin was scathing: 'Dr Salk, you should know better than to ask a question like that.'

Salk never forgave Sabin for putting him down so publically, and later said it was like 'being kicked in the teeth ... I could feel the resistance and hostility and the disapproval. I never attended a single one of those meetings afterward without that same feeling.'

Jonas Salk and Albert Sabin would compete fiercely and uncompromisingly for the rest of their lives. (Given their similar backgrounds, perhaps it was a form of sibling rivalry.) Salk worked to develop a 'killed vaccine', or inactivated polio vaccine (IPV), which had to be injected, whereas Sabin persisted with a 'live vaccine', using attenuated poliovirus that could be given by mouth, hence it was known as oral polio vaccine (OPV). Each was convinced his method was the best way to make a vaccine and neither would ever contemplate compromise or collaboration.

Salk's vaccine was the first to be tested on live subjects. Initially he tested it successfully on laboratory animals. Then in 1952 he injected 43 children at a 'home for crippled children', followed a few weeks later by children at a school for the 'retarded and feeble-minded'. Following this, Salk inoculated his wife and three sons with his vaccine.

Polio vaccine was at a critical point. Salk wanted to immunise people with his IPV to prevent cases of polio, but Sabin wanted the country to wait for OPV, which was still in development. Salk's critics accused him of being arrogant and glory-seeking.

In 1954, researchers in the United States, Canada and Finland conducted placebo-controlled field trials of IPV. Critics of the American trial said it was far too expensive, but FDR's March of Dimes funded the program. This became a huge bone of contention with Albert Sabin, who complained long and loud about favouritism.

The spectre of paralytic polio was so frightening that parents were desperate for their children to be part of the trial, and the authorities had to turn away many thousands who wanted to participate. The children in the trial were called Polio Pioneers and were given a special commemorative card: 420,000 children were injected with IPV and 200,000 control children with an inactive placebo. The trial was blind: neither the children's parents nor the doctors knew who had received which.

The eagerly anticipated results were announced at the University of Michigan at 10.20 am on 12 April 1955, the 10th anniversary of President Roosevelt's death. (In fact the results were already known: the report had been written four days earlier.)

There was an audience of 500 present in the auditorium, including over 100 reporters and 16 newsreel cameras, and more than 50,000 doctors were waiting for the result. All over the country, people tuned their radios and listened with bated breath.

The radio program *Voice of America* was set to transmit the results to Europe. Criminal trials paused to hear the news.

When a press release was issued, there was pandemonium. 'It works, it works!' shouted the reporters. They all tried to get their stories out at once. One climbed out of a window and took his fixed-line phone onto the roof so his message could be heard.

Department stores broadcast the news of the successful vaccine trial on speakers that had been set up specially. People danced in the streets in celebration. Church bells rang, sirens blasted.

More IPV was rapidly produced and the vaccine was licensed in the United States in 1955 with great fanfare. Elvis Presley was photographed receiving the vaccine in order to promote teenage immunisation.

But disaster was not far away. Two weeks after the launch, in April 1955, an infant was admitted to a Chicago hospital with flaccid paralysis of both legs. It was the first case in what came to be called the Cutter Incident, when more than 200,000 children were given a faulty vaccine, 40,000 of whom developed polio and 10 of whom died. (I discuss the incident in detail in Chapter 11.)

Within a month the first mass vaccination program against polio had stalled. This catastrophe at least had the benefit of stimulating the government to introduce strict regulations about vaccine manufacture. IPV was reintroduced after its safety had been assured, but not surprisingly people were hesitant and uptake was not at first as vigorous as previously.

Polio was a serious public health problem in the USSR, and in 1956 a delegation of Soviet scientists came to the United States to consult Jonas Salk on how to produce his vaccine. Albert Sabin seized the opportunity to invite the scientists to visit him in his laboratory at the University of Cincinnati, and he was rewarded with an invitation to go to the Soviet Union. Salk was also invited to visit, since Soviet scientists were having problems maintaining consistent efficacy of the Salk vaccine, but he decided not to accept.

Sabin spent a month in the USSR, and the Soviet scientists asked him to send them samples of his vaccine. On his return to America, Sabin asked the State Department for permission. The State Department approved the request, despite objections from the United States Defense Department, which was concerned that the live vaccine virus might be used for biological warfare.

The Soviet Union decided to buy Sabin's OPV, and in 1959 used it to immunise 10 million children. The results were so encouraging that the Soviet Health Ministry gave it to everyone under 20 years of age, so that 77 million people received OPV – far more than were given IPV during the trial of Salk's vaccine in the United States.

The Sabin OPV vaccine was released in the United States in 1961. The advantages of OPV are that it is much cheaper, it can be taken orally as drops (or in those days on a sugar lump), and it spreads from a baby's faeces to other members of the family, which immunises them (and shows we are nowhere near as clean as we think). The disadvantage (as mentioned before) is that OPV can become virulent and cause vaccine-associated paralytic poliomyelitis (VAPP), but that occurs only extraordinarily rarely: 1 case in every 2.5 million doses of OPV.

Although IPV had reduced the incidence of polio in the United States from 135 cases per million population in 1955 to 26 per million in 1961, OPV rapidly took over from IPV in the United States. The annual number of American cases of paralytic polio fell from about 20,000 in the 1950s to 2525 in 1960 and 61 in 1965.

Salk never accepted that immunising the population with OPV was a wise decision. In 1973 he wrote an opinion piece for the *New York Times* claiming that OPV was unsafe and advocating that the United States revert to using IPV.

It would be 24 years before the United States Government agreed that IPV should replace OPV in order to avoid cases of VAPP. Initially, in 1997, IPV was just used for the first dose of polio vaccine and OPV for all subsequent doses given in the United States, but since 2000, Jonas Salk's IPV has been used exclusively. In poorer countries, though, Sabin's OPV is generally preferred to IPV. As mentioned, OPV is a fraction of the price and can be given more easily; it also spreads to unimmunised relatives.

Although many pharmaceutical companies begged him to do so, Sabin refused to patent his vaccine. Albert Sabin could be grumpy and irritable but he was a highly ethical man. He believed polio vaccine should be available to all children, no matter how poor. He lived off his salary as a professor and never made a cent from his discovery.

The fame that came with polio vaccine took its toll on Jonas Salk. His wife, Donna, never came to terms with the effects that the publicity had on their relationship, and they divorced in 1968. Salk remarried two years later, to the artist Françoise Gilot (the mother of two children by Pablo Picasso). He spent his later years fighting for peace. He described war as the 'cancer of the world' and travelled the globe meeting leaders to call for ways to avoid war.

Salk and Sabin were American heroes and received many honours, though, perhaps surprisingly, not the Nobel Prize. Both OPV and IPV proved vital in combating one of humanity's most malignant infections, but ultimately perhaps it was their competitive insistence that their own vaccine was the only worthy option that deprived them of this honour. Maybe the Nobel Committee was worried they would squabble on the world stage.

'Polio endgame'

By the early 1980s, experts began to contemplate the possibility of global eradication of polio. The WHO's 1975 Expanded Programme on Immunization had increased world coverage, but there was still a long way to go.

Polio shares most of the characteristics that made it possible to eradicate smallpox. However, there are differences that make polio more difficult to eradicate. The symptoms of polio are highly variable and the diagnosis is rarely obvious at first. Most people transmitting polio are asymptomatic, so they cannot be identified. The poliovirus can exist for weeks or months under certain circumstances such as in untreated sewage, acting as a potential source of infection. There are also three strains of poliomyelitis – types 1, 2 and 3 – which all needed to be included in polio vaccines. For all these reasons, many experts thought poliomyelitis would never be eradicated. The WHO set out to prove them wrong.

The WHO introduced the Global Polio Eradication Initiative (GPEI) in 1988, with the aim of eradicating polio by the year 2000. Polio was endemic in 125 countries. In 1988, 350,000 cases of polio were reported globally – 1000 a day. There were four 'pillars' to the GPEI: better routine delivery of OPV; mass vaccination campaigns in countries or regions with high polio activity; better surveillance and testing of cases; and mop-up vaccination campaigns following any confirmed cases.

Early progress was impressive, although the target of global eradication by the year 2000 proved over-ambitious. Nevertheless, the number of countries where polio was endemic fell from 125 in 1988 to just 10 by 2001. The Americas were certified polio-free in 1994, the Western Pacific in 2000 and Europe in 2002. Type 2 poliovirus was eradicated from the world in 1999 and has not reappeared.

Progress in eradicating polio in Africa was initially slow. In 1990 there were some 4000 cases in Africa, by 1993 still 1000 in 34 countries. Football (soccer) is the most popular sport in Africa, and the WHO decided to initiate a campaign that pictured a soccer ball and had the theme 'Kick Polio Out of Africa'. The campaign was launched by Nelson Mandela on 2 August 1996. His opening words were: 'Africa is renowned for its beauty, its rich natural heritage and prolific resources – but equally, the image of its suffering children haunts the conscience of our continent and the world.'

By 2000 polio was circulating regularly in only three African countries: Egypt, Niger and Nigeria. The activity of the extremist group Boko Haram in northern Nigeria not only meant that polio persisted in that country, but also that it was occasionally reintroduced into other African countries such as Mali.

In 2010, to coincide with the 2010 Soccer World Cup in South Africa, Rotary launched a campaign targeting the 23 African countries where polio was still a threat. Bishop Desmond Tutu was one of several leading African figures who signed a soccer ball that was taken around and exhibited in the target countries. Children were encouraged to find Bishop Tutu's signature on the ball.

Nigeria reported no cases of polio in 2015, four cases in 2016, and none since. Polio is about to be kicked out of Africa forever.

India has also proved a particular challenge. From the 1970s until the early 1990s there were 200,000 to 400,000 new cases there each year. Between 500 and 1000 children were paralysed by polio every day. By 1990, when 80% of the population had received three doses of OPV, the incidence was beginning to fall.

In 1995, India held its first National Immunization Day, when an astonishing 8 million children received oral polio vaccine at fixed booths around the country. From 2004, 10 of these 'pulse polio campaigns' were conducted every year, and virtually every child in India was tracked down and vaccinated.

In 1990, there had been over 3000 new cases of polio in New Delhi alone. In 2009 almost half the new cases of polio in the world were still occurring in India, and eradication seemed a distant if not impossible goal. There were pockets of persistent infection, notably among children in poor, isolated provinces like Uttar Pradesh. Polio workers tried to reach these children by going house to house. In 2011, after using over a million vaccinators to reach remote areas, polio was eliminated from the whole of India. The last known victim was 18-month-old Rukhsar Khatoon from West Bengal. As Bill Gates said without hyperbole: 'India's achievement is one of the most impressive accomplishments in global health, ever.'

The crippling nature of polio and the drama of its eradication is illustrated by the story of Dr Mathew Varghese, whom Bill Gates visited in his hospital. Dr Varghese is an orthopaedic surgeon who for years ran the only dedicated polio ward in India, at St Stephen's Hospital in New Delhi. The ward was supported financially by Rotary. Dr Varghese accepted every patient who came to see him, whether or not they could afford to pay for treatment. He performed surgery on afflicted children who could only crawl, enabling them to stand, and later to walk using braces or callipers. Dr Varghese treated children with one leg shortened from polio using leg-lengthening surgery, often allowing them to discard crutches and walk unaided. When polio was eliminated, Dr Varghese was thrilled to be able to close his polio ward.

Another polio hero was the late Brazilian epidemiologist Ciro de Quadros (1940–2014), who was Director of PAHO, the Pan American Health Organization. From 1985, de Quadros sent teams of polio workers to the most remote and war-ravaged regions of Latin America. His health workers recruited local volunteers and organised mass immunisations of children under five to coincide with local religious festivals. In war-torn El Salvador and Guatemala they negotiated 'tranquillity days', 24-hour ceasefires between rebel and government forces, to allow health workers to immunise children. They could not persuade the Shining Path guerrillas in Peru to cooperate, so they worked around the rebel-held areas and went back to mop up when the battlelines shifted. The last reported case of polio in Latin America was in Pichinaki, Peru, in 1991.

DA Henderson, leader of the WHO's Smallpox Eradication Unit, recognised de Quadros as being not only a great epidemiologist but also a fearless and inspirational leader. DA had recruited de Quadros in 1971 to help eliminate smallpox in Ethiopia, which was fighting a prolonged civil war with Eritrea. Six of de Quadros's teams were kidnapped by armed rebels, who also commandeered a United Nations helicopter with its pilot on board. De Quadros helped negotiate the return of the health workers and the pilot, all of whom resumed their work in the field. DA Henderson later said: 'That's a measure of the dedication he inspired. Even that helicopter pilot vaccinated the rebels who held him.'

Progress in eradicating polio stagnated in the early years of the new millennium in countries where there was conflict, political instability, limited access to remote regions, and poor healthcare systems. Immunisation levels fell in the tribal areas of Pakistan in 2009 when an influential local Muslim cleric, Maulana Fazlullah, launched a campaign against polio vaccination. His daily sermons, broadcast on radio and through mosque loudspeakers, denounced it as an American plot to sterilise Muslim children and reduce the Pakistani population. The Pakistani Taliban leadership campaigned against the vaccination programs, and appeared to target female healthcare workers.

Conspiracy theories about vaccination were given huge momentum in July 2012, when it was discovered that the United States Central Intelligence Agency (CIA) had recruited the assistance of a Pakistani doctor, Shakil Afridi, in mounting a fake hepatitis B immunisation campaign, in order to track down Osama bin Laden, former leader of al-Qaeda. Immunisation advocates were horrified that the CIA would jeopardise trust in immunisation in such a cynical fashion. The CIA argued that the ends justified the means. The relatives of immunisation workers killed in Pakistan by the Taliban would probably disagree.

Salma Farooqi, 30 years old, a dedicated nurse and mother of five, was famous for years of tireless work immunising children against polio in the town of Peshawar near the Khyber Pass. At 1am on Sunday 23 March 2014, armed men stormed her house, tied up other members of her family and took her away. The next day her body was found in a field 4 kilometres away. She had been tortured and repeatedly shot.

Over the previous two years, more than 30 Pakistani vaccinators had been killed by the Taliban. Some 100,000 of the polio vaccinators were teenage girls and young women, Pakistan's 'Lady Health Workers'. Salma knew the risks, which makes her extraordinary courage all the more praiseworthy.

In Nigeria, too, polio vaccinators have been targeted and killed by extremists. On 8 February 2013, nine young women giving polio vaccinations were killed by gunmen in an area in Northern Nigeria known to have been targeted by Boko Haram. Just days afterwards, a controversial Islamic leader claimed that polio was caused by contaminated medicine.

Yet even in such war-ravaged countries there are glimmers of hope. From January 2016, the Taliban blocked polio immunisation in Kunduz province in northern Afghanistan, saying they would only resume immunisation if the WHO built a clinic in the remote Char Data district to treat civilians and soldiers wounded by American bombs. The WHO does not run trauma clinics and was unable to comply, but this left 170,000 children in Kunduz province unimmunised.

In April 2017, elders in a remote village in the region were devastated when a 14-month-old became paralysed by polio. She was the third child in the village to be paralysed that year. In desperation the elders appealed to the Taliban.

Qari Bashir, the province's Taliban health chief, was sceptical that the WHO truly had the interests of Afghan children at heart. 'Every day the Americans are bombing Afghan children. I don't think that [the little girl's paralysis] was so important to them,' he said.

Amazingly, though, Bashir listened to the elders' plea, took pity on them and allowed polio immunisation to resume. It is a poignant illustration of how humanity can trump politics.

The strategy the WHO calls the 'polio endgame' has not proved easy. We have already heard that OPV vaccine can very rarely (1 in 2.5 million doses) cause vaccine-associated paralytic poliomyelitis (VAPP). In a poorly immunised population the VAPP strain can spread to unimmunised children and adults and cause a small cluster of cases. This is called circulating vaccine-derived poliovirus, or cVDPV. To eradicate polio completely – both wild-type and vaccine-derived polioviruses – the world will need to change from OPV to IPV, because IPV cannot lead to cVDPV.

By the end of 2016, 173 countries were using IPV in their routine immunisation schedules. There has been great pressure on the supply of IPV: it costs more, and it has to be delivered via injection by qualified health staff.

Yet perseverance is vital. Modelling studies estimate that if we stopped immunising against polio now, there would be 200,000 new cases within five years.

Polio eradication is tantalisingly close. When it is achieved, it will be one of the greatest human achievements, to be placed alongside the elimination of smallpox with justifiable pride.

CHAPTER 5

Tuberculosis, the great equaliser

Yet the captain of all these men of death that came against him to take him away was the consumption, for it was that that brought him down to the grave.

The Life and Death of Mr Badman, John Bunyan (1626–1688)

For some inexplicable reason, tuberculosis (TB) is often linked with romance. Lord Byron is partly to blame; he was an incurable romantic who had fantasies of dying slowly from tuberculosis in order to impress his many mistresses.

Henry David Thoreau – American poet, philosopher, emancipist and eternal optimist – caught TB when he was 18 and it plagued him on and off until he died from it in 1862, aged 44. Yet he once wrote: 'Decay and disease are often beautiful, like the pearly tear of the shellfish and the hectic glow of consumption.'

Consumption is an old name for tuberculosis, deriving from the fact that it is a slow disease that causes the sufferer to become thinner and thinner, as if consumed by it. The name suggests a dallying, dreamlike death, rather than the true picture of terminal tuberculosis, which is a death characterised by starvation, weakness, exhaustion and depression. Other archaic names for tuberculosis were 'the phthisis', which means wasting, and 'the white plague' and 'the white death', so called because of the pallor caused by anaemia due to chronic tuberculosis.

Tuberculosis is and always was a horrible, debilitating disease, and it has killed more people than any other infectious disease in history. It has affected the world in myriad ways, leaving its imprint on humankind in real life, in literature, in the visual arts and in science. In *Nicholas Nickleby*, Charles Dickens called it 'a dread disease' that 'medicine never cured' and 'wealth never warded off', an illness 'in which death and life are so strangely blended, that death takes the glow and hue of life, and life the gaunt and grisly form of death'.

Wealth never warded it off because TB was no respecter of class; most other infections were diseases of the poor, but TB was feared by everyone because it could kill anyone. When American author Susan Sontag was being treated for cancer she wrote a book, *Illness as Metaphor*, in which she likened 20th-century cancer to 19th-century tuberculosis. Both are 'obscene in the original meaning of that word: ill-omened, abominable, repugnant to the senses'. As Siddhartha Mukherjee wrote when comparing TB and cancer in his wonderful book *The Emperor of All Maladies*, 'Both drain vitality: both stretch out the encounter with death; in both cases, dying, even more than death, defines the illness.'

John Keats might have been a romantic poet, but TB wrecked his short life. His father died after a fall from a horse when Keats was eight, then his mother died from TB when Keats was 14. After that his grandmother looked after John and his three younger siblings. Keats studied medicine at Guy's Hospital in London, but found that his studies got in the way of his first love, writing poetry. So he dropped out of medical school and pursued a career as a writer. John's favourite brother, George, migrated to the United States, but his investments failed and both he and his wife Georgina died penniless and racked with tuberculosis. John nursed his other dying brother, Tom, until Tom too succumbed to tuberculosis at age 19.

In 1820 John Keats started coughing and getting weaker and weaker. At first he was brave. In his famous poem 'Ode to a Nightingale', which he composed while reclining in the shade of a plum tree in his Hampstead garden, he wrote:

> Darkling I listen; and, for many a time
> Call'd him soft names in many a mused rhyme
> To take into the air my quiet breath;
> I have been half in love with easeful Death.

Yet easeful death did not come easily. Twice John Keats coughed up huge volumes of blood. He was persuaded that Italy would be good for his health and moved to an apartment next to the Spanish Steps in Rome. On the sea voyage and again in Rome he tried to persuade his dear friend and travelling companion Joseph Severn to give him laudanum (opium) – supposedly to relieve his pain, but in truth to end his suffering. Keats would sometimes cry when he woke up and found he was still alive. He often asked: 'How long is this posthumous existence of mine to go on?'

Finally Severn wrote: 'Keats raves till I am in a complete tremble for him ... I lifted him up in my arms. The phlegm seem'd boiling in his throat, and increased until eleven, when he gradually sank into death, so quiet, that I still thought he slept.'

John Keats was just 25. He was buried in Rome, and at his last request was placed under a tombstone with no name or date, only the words 'Here lies One whose Name was writ in Water.' There is nothing romantic about tuberculosis.

Still, operas continued to romanticise tuberculosis in the mid-19th century, until realism eventually held sway. In Giuseppe Verdi's *La Traviata*, which premiered in 1853, the wealthy heroine Violetta becomes more sensitive after catching TB. By 1896, in contrast, Giacomo Puccini portrays tuberculosis as a disease of poverty in *La Bohème*. His heroine Mimi dies destitute. Mimi's lover Rodolfo abandons her, probably from fear of catching her infection: 'Amo Mimi, ma ho paura' ('I love Mimi, but I am afraid'), he sings. But this is opera, and he returns to her, only to find her dying with her tiny hands frozen. There is romance and tragedy in *La Bohème*, but the tuberculosis is part of the tragedy, not of the romance. Chopin aged 39, Purcell at 36, Paganini at 58 and Stravinsky at 89 – all died of tuberculosis. In the 19th century, tuberculosis was the main killer in Europe and the United States: every year 1 in every 40 people died from TB, the white plague.

The origins of tuberculosis

Tuberculosis is as old as humanity. For a while experts thought TB originated less than 6000 years ago. However, more recent genetic analysis of strains of TB suggests the organism first emerged in humans in Africa around 70,000 years ago, was carried by people who migrated into Europe and Asia, and began to infect people during the Neolithic period (roughly 10,000 to 2000 BC). It wasn't until large numbers of people began living in close proximity, however, that it spread widely.

In an extraordinary multidisciplinary research paper published in 2016, Australian authors hypothesised, on the basis of mathematical modelling, epidemiology, evolutionary genetics and paleoanthropology, that TB might have emerged at the time when humans learned how to control the use of fire. They argued that controlled use of fire altered lifestyle and provided ideal conditions for *Mycobacterium tuberculosis* to evolve because from then on people would huddle together round fires, often in caves, and cough on each other.

One of the fascinating things about human infectious diseases is that many of them come from animals or birds. Influenza originated in birds and pigs before infecting humans. The hepatitis B, polio and HIV viruses all derived from viruses that infected monkeys and apes before reaching humans. Measles virus came from the rinderpest virus of cattle. But TB is unusual, in that genetic studies suggest it emerged in humans *before* it appeared in any animals, and spread later to cows, and even later to animals like badgers when they came into close contact with cattle.

Mycobacterium tuberculosis is usually caught through being inhaled. It can cause severe lung disease, but it can also spread to the lymph nodes. The commonest site for enlarged lymph nodes is the neck. Indeed, the name tuberculosis (first used in 1839) comes from the Latin *tuberculum*, meaning a small tuber, because infected neck nodes were thought to look like small vegetable tubers.

It has long been recognised that people could develop enlarged, rubbery, painless swellings in the neck that could rupture, discharging blood-stained pus and leaving the neck chronically scarred by festering sores. This condition was known in the Middle Ages as 'scrofula', from the Latin *scrofa*, a breeding sow. (The link between a sow and TB is puzzling. Some point out that *scrofula* means 'female piglet', but pigs do not get TB. My own suspicion is that it gained this name because the udders of a breeding sow lie in a line that resembles the line of enlarged neck nodes in TB.)

Another name for scrofula was the 'king's evil', and it was said in centuries past that it could be cured by royal touch, supposedly a divine gift from God. The practice began in France, persisting from King Clovis in the fifth century to Louis XVI, who was beheaded during the French Revolution in 1793. It was said that Henry IV (reigned 1589–1610) would touch and heal as many as 1500 scrofulous citizens at a sitting.

In England, the tradition started with Edward the Confessor in the 11th century and lasted until the accession of the more down-to-earth Hanoverians in the 18th century. The English king or queen would not only touch the sufferer, but also give them a gold coin called an angel, which was actually quite valuable. William Shakespeare wrote *Macbeth* for King James I, who had revised the lapsed practice of the royal touch. In Act IV, Scene 3, Malcolm says: 'A most miraculous work in this good King, which often since my here-remain in England, I have seen him do. How he solicits heaven, Himself best knows; but strangely-visited people all swollen and ulcerous, pitiful to the eye, the mere despair of surgery he cures.'

The royal touch may seem rather bizarre and improbable now, but hindsight is a wonderful thing, and many of *our* current ceremonies will surely amaze our descendants.

TB can spread in the bloodstream to the bones, liver and spleen. The bones of the spine can become permanently bent forward in what is called a gibbus deformity (*gibbus* is Latin for 'hump'.) Some 5000-year-old Egyptian mummies show this same classic symptom of TB in their vertebral column, causing their spine to bend forward at a sharp angle like the broken branch of a tree. The Hunchback of Nôtre Dame probably had TB of the spine. Most worryingly, TB can reach the lining of the brain called the meninges and cause meningitis, a disease that kills many of its victims and often leaves survivors brain-damaged (as we'll see in Chapter 7).

People can develop TB if they drink milk from cows infected with *Mycobacterium bovis*, which causes bovine TB. In this case they usually get TB of the intestines, which can also spread to the rest of the body. In the 1890s, Finland started testing cattle for TB using a technique called tuberculin testing, and managed to eliminate bovine TB. All industrialised countries now routinely use tuberculin testing on cattle and pasteurise cow's milk, so catching TB from cow's milk is almost unheard of in these parts of the world. However, TB can still be acquired from drinking unpasteurised milk from cows, sheep or goats in resource-poor countries.

A cure for tuberculosis

Before the 20th century, prevention of human TB was the only option. In 1882, the German physician and microbiologist Robert Koch was able to grow the organism that causes tuberculosis.

With characteristic modesty, he called tuberculosis 'Koch's disease' and the organism 'Koch's bacillus'.

Around the same time, it was confirmed that TB was contagious. Australia and other Western countries instituted public health campaigns against spitting on trams and trains and in the streets, because sputum could contain tubercle bacilli. TB affected fashion too. Reports that the bacilli could be caught in long skirts encouraged the raising of hemlines – a cartoon called 'The Trailing Skirt: Death Loves a Shining Mark' appeared in an American magazine, *Puck*, in 1900, showing a maid shaking off clouds of germs from her lady's skirt, watched by a scythe-bearing Death. Heavy-boned Victorian corsets, thought to exacerbate tuberculosis by preventing breathing and cutting off circulation, were replaced by elastic 'health corsets'. Men shaved off beards and moustaches that might harbour germs.

After World War I, French scientists Albert Calmette and Camille Guérin developed a vaccine using *Mycobacterium bovis*, the organism that causes TB in cows. Between 1908 and 1921, they cultured and recultured the organism 230 times to attenuate it, a technique called 'passaging'. Their vaccine was first used in 1921 and is named, in their honour, the Bacille Calmette-Guérin or BCG vaccine. It is the oldest vaccine still in use today.

Confidence in the safety and efficacy of injected BCG vaccine was bolstered by large, carefully conducted clinical trials. The first mass BCG immunisation campaign was started in Poland in 1948.

However, the effectiveness of BCG vaccine varies. For some unknown reason, it is more effective nearer the equator and less effective in East Asia. Overall, BCG prevents about 70% of TB cases, although the efficacy varies from zero (usually where the vaccine was not preserved properly) to 80% in different studies.

It is more effective in preventing severe than mild TB disease: it is 90% effective in preventing TB meningitis and disseminated TB. The vaccine is by no means perfect, and we would love a better TB vaccine, especially one that would prevent TB circulating. The protection offered by BCG vaccine is a whole lot better than none, though, and BCG vaccine is still used in developing countries worldwide. However, the lack of a vaccine that prevents transmission has necessitated the use of antibiotics in the treatment of TB. These have to be given for months, which has contributed to the worrying emergence of antibiotic-resistant tuberculosis.

From the 1880s, invasive lung surgery was used to treat TB, but it was never subjected to trials to see if it worked. It almost certainly did no good. Often doctors would deliberately collapse one lung. One technique was to pump oxygen or nitrogen into the chest cavity under pressure. Another operation was thoracoplasty, which involved removing part of the rib-cage so the chest wall collapsed. Mycobacteria need oxygen to survive, so the aim was to deprive them of oxygen, but the surgery was deforming and sometimes fatal; the 'cure' may well have been worse than the disease. Over the next 25 years, 100,000 patients had a lung collapsed, until the practice fell out of favour.

In the 1930s and 1940s, a treatment known as phrenic paralysis came into fashion. This involved crushing the phrenic nerve, which runs beside the lung and causes the diaphragm to work, so that diaphragm would be paralysed and the lung on that side would not inflate or deflate until the nerve healed. The apparent rationale was that if the lung did not inflate, the TB organisms would be deprived of oxygen. The trouble was, the poor patient was also deprived of oxygen.

Improved sanitation and cleaner water, then the development of BCG vaccine, saw a slow decline in TB, but it would take the advent of effective antibiotics in the 1940s for TB to all but disappear from Western countries within a few years.

As scientists worked to develop an antibiotic cure, tuberculosis was the focus of the first ever large-scale double-blind randomised controlled trials. 'Double blind' means that neither the participants nor the researchers know which treatment the patient has received until the trial is completed. 'Randomised' means the patients are randomly assigned to one or the other treatment, for example by being given a vial with a coded number, with the code only broken at the end of the trial. The trial is 'controlled' because the patient is given either the new treatment or an alternative, and the patients receiving the alternative act as a 'control' for the active vaccine; the vaccine recipients can then be compared with the controls.

Scientists had long known it was wise to include a control group in trials: if the control group got better just as quickly as treated patients, the treatment had done nothing, except perhaps cause side effects. One of the first controlled clinical trials was carried out by James Lind, a medical apprentice from Edinburgh. He joined the Royal Navy as a surgeon's mate in the late 1730s. In 1747, on board HMS *Salisbury*, he divided 12 men suffering from similar symptoms of scurvy into six pairs and treated each pair with a different popular remedy: a quart of cider; elixir of vitriol; half a pint of sea-water; a paste made of garlic, mustard seed, horseradish, balsam of Peru (a mix of cinnamon and vanilla) and gum myrrh; vinegar; and finally citrus fruits (specifically two oranges and one lemon). By the end of the week, the two men who received citrus fruits had recovered sufficiently to nurse the others.

While Lind's was a successful controlled trial, trials such as this, where it is known which treatment the patient is getting, are susceptible to bias. Well-meaning researchers can inadvertently affect the results, for example by making sure the sickest patients receive the treatment they think is most likely to work. This tendency to bias is only human.

In the United Kingdom in the 1940s, a new antibiotic, streptomycin, was found to be active against tuberculosis in the laboratory. It was in short supply. The British Medical Research Council elicited the help of a statistician, Bradford Hill, who pointed out that the scarcity of streptomycin ethically justified trials in which only half the patients received the drug.

Hill felt that doctors could not be trusted to avoid bias, conscious or unconscious, and to guard against this he proposed randomly determining which patients would receive streptomycin and which would not. For the latter group, he suggested using a disguised placebo instead of no treatment. This meant that both patients and doctors were 'blinded' as to which treatment had been given.

The trial clearly showed that patients given streptomycin fared better. Streptomycin caused deafness and was later superseded by less toxic drugs, but Bradford Hill's scientific method has survived. He was deservedly knighted for his contribution to science.

Tuberculosis today

Almost every industrialised country used to give routine BCG immunisation to children. But tuberculosis is rare in industrialised countries nowadays, not because of antibiotics or BCG vaccine but because of improved living standards. As TB disappeared from the Western world, BCG immunisation programs were stopped, and now countries like Australia only recommend BCG vaccine for people who are in contact with a person with infectious TB, or people planning to live in countries with a high incidence of TB. BCG vaccine is no longer given orally but intradermally – as an injection into the skin that is slowly absorbed.

In developing countries, however, BCG vaccine is still given routinely to newborns and still saves lives. Since 1974, BCG has been part of the WHO's Expanded Programme on Immunization in all countries with a high incidence of TB disease.

Tuberculosis remains a major problem in these countries. In 1990, I was invited to teach in Kota Bharu in Northern Malaysia. When I visited the colourful local market, I was shocked to see two hunchbacked children of perhaps seven or eight, begging among the stalls. Their spines were permanently deformed by tuberculosis.

TB is still the number-one killer among infectious diseases (though almost exclusively in developing countries). Yet not everyone exposed to TB becomes infected, and not everyone infected becomes ill with disease. *Mycobacterium tuberculosis* is a very slow-growing organism that can remain hidden (latent) in the body for years. If a child becomes ill with tuberculosis in an industrialised country nowadays, they have usually been infected by a parent who was born in a poor overseas country or the child has spent a prolonged time overseas. An adult in an industrialised country who develops TB was usually born in a poor country and infected with TB as a child, and the TB has come back many years later. We have effective antibiotics against TB, but have to use three or four at once to stop resistance to the drugs developing. Worldwide there is an increasing problem with strains of TB becoming resistant to a number of antibiotics (multi-resistant TB), necessitating the use of more experimental and more toxic antibiotics.

A third of the current world population has been infected with TB. Less than 10% of them will develop the disease at some time in their lives. The WHO reported that in 2016 more than 10 million people globally became ill from TB and 1.3 million died. More than 95% of them lived in low- and middle-income countries and over half of them in just five countries: China, India, Indonesia, Pakistan and the Philippines.

Tuberculosis is no longer the great killer that it was in the 19th century, and it is a tribute to the human immune system that more than 90% of people infected with tuberculosis will manage to keep the disease forever at bay. Nevertheless, tuberculosis remains a festering human health problem, and the development of more effective vaccines against tuberculosis is one of science's top priorities.

CHAPTER 6

Diphtheria, the scourge of childhood

Memories are short. People nowadays worry more about whether vaccines are safe than about what infections their child might catch if unimmunised. Yet even within living memory, before almost any vaccines existed, the story was so different.

A close friend and colleague used to visit Deniliquin in country New South Wales as a child. He was an inquisitive boy and asked why there were six white posts clustered together in a distant field. They marked the spot where the three children of the neighbouring farmer had been buried, at a safe distance from any human habitation, after they all died from diphtheria. In the decade from 1926 to 1935, more than 4000 children died from diphtheria in Australia.

Samuel Clemens had been a printer's apprentice, a steamboat pilot on the Mississippi River, a prospector who found no gold, and a Confederate soldier who never fought in a battle, but in

1861 he headed west in search of adventure. There he wrote about his experiences and also met Olivia (Livy) Langdon, the love of his life. He courted her for 17 months, and finally they married. Clemens's first book, *The Innocents Abroad*, was a great success. He published it under the nom de plume of Mark Twain (Twain means two; 'Mark twain' would have been shouted out on the steamboat when the plumb-line showed a depth of 2 fathoms).

Yet tragedy soon struck Sam and Livy. In 1872, their first son, 17-month-old Langdon, contracted diphtheria, which choked him to death. He died in his mother's arms. Clemens always blamed himself for Langdon's death, saying Langdon caught a chill in his carriage when Clemens let slip the blanket covering him.

We now know that catching a chill is *not* the cause of diphtheria. Clemens was innocent of all blame. Had Langdon been born less than a century later, in the golden age of immunisation, he would never have caught diphtheria and might even have become a great writer like his father.

All about diphtheria

Diphtheria is a dreaded disease that hits communities in epidemic waves and used to be called 'the scourge of childhood'. The 16th century Belgian physician Joost van Lom (also known as Jodocus Lommius) wrote of the disease:

> The patient is racked with pain, labours under a violent fever and dreads suffocation. The mouth is open wide, gasps for cool air and discharges a frothy saliva. The tongue hangs out and is frequently agitated like that of over-ridden horses. The liquor drunk returns through the nostrils, the lips become

livid, and the neck is rendered rigid ... on account of the
violence of the suffocation, the patient neither knows what
he hears or says or does, till at last being seized with syncope
[fainting] he dies.

British bacteriologist Frederick Andrewes wrote in 1923, 'The
manner of death is described as most piteous, for the breath had
a putrefactive odour so that the patients could not endure the
smell of themselves.' Sometimes a terrified child's neck will swell
up with inflammation to give a 'bull neck' appearance.

Diphtheria was described clinically by the great Greek
physician Hippocrates, and its name comes from the Greek word
for a leather hide, because of the thick membrane that forms and
sticks to the throat, choking the victim to death. A 17th century
Spanish physician, Juan de Villareal, described the membrane
as having the consistency of wet leather or wet parchment. In
Spain, 1613 is still known as *El año de los garrotillos*, the year of
strangulations, because of a devastating outbreak of diphtheria
that killed thousands of children and young adults. (The Spanish
used to execute prisoners by garrotting, so they were experts
on the symptoms.) Diphtheria spread from Spain, where it was
known as 'the strangler', to Italy, where it was called 'the gullet
disease'.

To perform a tracheostomy, making a hole in the windpipe
while the patient is still awake, was the only hope of survival
for many children and young adults suffocating to death from
diphtheria. The first person to perform a tracheostomy for
diphtheria was the same man who gave diphtheria its name, the
famous French physician Pierre Fidèle Bretonneau of Tours. That
Bretonneau had made two unsuccessful attempts at tracheostomy

for diphtheria before succeeding is less well remembered. He performed the first successful tracheostomy in 1825, on four-year-old Elisabeth de Puységur. She survived and became the Comtesse de Billy, which success did as much for his reputation as the 540-page treatise he wrote on diphtheria.

Finding a vaccine

In 1884, German microbiologists Edwin Klebs and Friedrich Löffler described the organism *Corynebacterium diphtheriae* (sometimes called the Klebs-Löffler bacillus), which was the cause of the diphtheria that killed Langdon Clemens and millions of other children.

In 1888, Louis Pasteur's long-suffering colleague Emile Roux and Swiss microbiologist Alexandre Yersin showed that the organisms causing diphtheria produce a toxin (poisonous substance) that could cause disease at a distant site. Many patients died from diphtheria as the toxin spread in the bloodstream, poisoning the heart, which failed, and their nerves, which paralysed them.

A toxoid is a toxin that has been weakened with heat or chemicals. The diphtheria vaccine we have used for almost a century is made by modifying diphtheria toxin using the chemical formaldehyde. Thus, the discovery of diphtheria toxin was a critical piece of research.

The first diphtheria toxoid vaccine suitable for widespread use in humans was developed in 1923. Before that time the most effective treatment for people with diphtheria was to use an antitoxin. The principle of an antitoxin is that if you can make an animal immune by injecting it with the toxin from the organism, then you can use the animal's serum (blood plasma) as an antitoxin.

We now know that this is possible because the animal produces antibodies to protect itself, and injecting those antibodies provides the human with passive protection – passive immunisation as it's known. This is a different process from most modern immunisations, which use a vaccine to stimulate a lasting immune response for future protection (active immunisation).

The first diphtheria antitoxin was developed in 1890 in Berlin by Kitasato Shibasaburō, a baron of the Empire of Japan, and Emil von Behring, later a professor of hygienics. They showed that if they heated diphtheria toxin and injected it into guinea-pigs, the guinea-pigs were protected against diphtheria infection and against further injections of diphtheria toxin. Moreover, they could cure a guinea-pig suffering from diphtheria by injecting serum from a guinea-pig immunised with heated toxin (toxoid).

They had in fact discovered the principle of making a toxoid vaccine and, had they decided to take that route, could have developed a diphtheria toxoid vaccine before 1923. However, that is easy to say with hindsight. At the time, they followed a different route, which was to mass-produce antitoxin for passive immunisation.

A guinea-pig doesn't contain much serum, so they thought bigger. They had problems immunising cows and sheep, but horses proved a success. When given repeated doses of the toxin they developed antibodies, and could be bled to yield a potent antitoxin. Horse antiserum could cause severe allergic reactions and even anaphylaxis, but it saved many thousands of children and adults from dying of diphtheria.

Emil von Behring became a national hero, and was called 'the saviour of children', ennobled into the Prussian nobility, and awarded the first ever Nobel Prize in Physiology or Medicine. Kitasato Shibasaburō was nominated for the Nobel Prize but got nothing. Either he was just not pushy enough or he was plumb unlucky.

On a sour note, von Behring never acknowledged the contribution of a major collaborator, Paul Ehrlich, a German scientist. Ehrlich always felt von Behring cheated him out of the considerable rewards that resulted from developing diphtheria antiserum.

Although diphtheria antitoxin produced in horses reduced mortality, a sceptic could say it was shutting the stable door after the horse had bolted. It only worked once a child had diphtheria, and did nothing to prevent children from catching the disease or spreading it to other children. We know prevention is better than cure. The situation came to a head in the United States in 1921, when there were an unprecedented 206,000 cases of diphtheria, causing 15,520 deaths.

William H Park was a bacteriologist who headed the laboratory at the New York City Board of Health. Park was an innovator who, although best known for his pioneering work on diphtheria, published research on many other childhood infections.

Park had long been an advocate of diphtheria antitoxin, and initiated an ambitious diphtheria antitoxin program in New York schools from 1918. In the space of 15 years, the City of New York administered 500,000 doses. The number of deaths each year from diphtheria fell from 800 in 1920, to 416 in 1929, and 198 in 1930.

Meanwhile, in 1923, AT Glenny and Barbara Hopkins from the Wellcome Research Laboratories in Beckenham, Kent, published a seminal paper, 'Diphtheria Toxoid as an Immunising Agent'. They not only showed that diphtheria toxoid induced a much stronger immune response than antitoxin, but also that a small amount of alum (aluminium salts) could be added to act as an adjuvant (a substance that improves the immune response – from the Latin for 'help').

Park was impressed, and started to use a diphtheria toxoid vaccine made in the United States that was based on Glenny and Hopkins's vaccine. Park performed studies comparing children's antibody responses to three different vaccines. He found that antibodies were produced by 90% of children given diphtheria antitoxin, 93.7% given diphtheria toxoid without alum and 98.2% given diphtheria toxoid with alum. Park's work was an important step in proving that diphtheria toxoid with an alum adjuvant was the most protective vaccine. He also showed it was extremely safe.

The particular strain of *Corynebacterium diphtheriae* most often used to make contemporary diphtheria toxoid vaccines was discovered by Dr Anna Williams, who worked in Dr Park's laboratory. A biography written about Park is called *The Man Who Lived for Tomorrow*. Park's tomorrow is our today. The diphtheria toxoid his laboratory produced is the basis for all modern diphtheria vaccines.

Australia introduced school-based diphtheria vaccination programs in 1932 and routine infant immunisation in 1940, which led to a rapid and sustained reduction in diphtheria. A similar pattern was seen throughout the United States, Canada and Western Europe. In the United States from 2004 until the end of 2017, there were only two cases of diphtheria throughout the entire country.

Diphtheria today

We may reassure ourselves and say: 'Diphtheria has gone. It won't ever come back to a safe country like ours.' However, the organism that causes diphtheria, *Corynebacterium diphtheriae*, has not gone away. It still circulates in the throats of healthy children and adults. Being immunised protects us against developing the disease, even if the organism infects us. But if we stop immunising, even in rich countries where children are healthy and well fed, diphtheria will return.

This was illustrated with a vengeance in Russia and surrounding countries as recently as the 1990s. The Soviet Union introduced routine childhood immunisation in the late 1950s, but poor health infrastructure meant that cases of diphtheria still occurred in the 1970s and 1980s. After the Soviet Union was dissolved in 1991, health services broke down and there were massive diphtheria outbreaks in Moscow and St Petersburg, as well as in the Ukraine and Belarus. Between 1991 and 1996, over 140,000 people fell ill and more than 4000 died. Almost all the cases occurred in unvaccinated children and adults. The epidemic was eventually halted by producing more diphtheria vaccine and by improving public health infrastructure.

Vaccine opponents often claim that infectious diseases were disappearing before immunisations were introduced, due to improved living standards, and that all you need to avoid infection is good nutrition and tender loving care. Yet these victims were not starving or even hungry; they simply became infected with the organism that causes diphtheria. This sad saga was a lesson, if one was needed, of the value of immunisation, the rapidity with which previously feared diseases can return if we stop immunising, and the fact that these diseases cannot be prevented by adequate nutrition alone.

Thanks to immunisation, no Australian child has died from diphtheria for more than 25 years. But there is no reason to be blasé. If you think you are safe if you remain unimmunised in Australia, think again. Australia has had an average of five cases per year in the last four years, after only 13 in the previous 23 years.

The most recent Australian to catch diphtheria, in January 2018, was a previously healthy unimmunised 27-year-old man from Cairns in Far North Queensland. He died in Brisbane Hospital.

We do not know whether this recent rise in diphtheria in Australia is due to people who catch diphtheria overseas then bring it home to infect others, or whether it is because unimmunised people are being infected with home-grown bugs. But the message is clear: diphtheria has not gone away. If you want to be protected against it, get yourself and your children immunised.

CHAPTER 7

The golden age of immunisation

Nowadays we take our children to the doctor for their routine immunisations with no thought of what went into making those vaccines. Routine childhood vaccination against diphtheria and tetanus commenced in the early 1940s in Australia. By 1949, pertussis vaccine had been added to create a 'triple vaccine' called DTP (diphtheria-tetanus-pertussis), with the aim of reducing the number of injections a child receives.

When my children were infants in the 1980s, they were injected with three doses of the DTP triple vaccine, and ate three doses of OPV polio vaccine on a sugar lump. At 15 months they got measles vaccine.

My first grandson, born in 2014, was given three doses of a hexavalent or six-in-one vaccine as a baby that protected him against diphtheria, tetanus and pertussis, as well as *Haemophilus influenzae* type b (Hib) – previously the most common cause of childhood meningitis – and hepatitis B. The vaccine included inactivated polio vaccine (IPV) instead of giving it by mouth. However, he did receive rotavirus vaccine by mouth to protect him against the nastiest cause of infant gastroenteritis. Later he received MMR vaccine against measles, mumps and rubella, and immunisations to protect him against varicella (chickenpox), meningococcus – which causes meningitis – and pneumococcus – which causes pneumonia or meningitis. When he is in secondary school he will receive human papillomavirus vaccine (HPV) to stop him from getting cancer of the penis or anus and to help protect any future female sexual partners against cancer of the cervix. My grandson will be protected against 14 diseases altogether, compared with the five his mother was vaccinated against. That is a huge step forward.

We owe a debt of gratitude to the scientists of the late 19th and early 20th centuries who helped usher in the golden age of immunisation that has now lasted the best part of a century.

As we saw in Chapter 2, smallpox vaccine was the first vaccine to be used to immunise whole populations, starting around 1800. However, smallpox vaccine had been developed because of the similarity between the highly pathogenic smallpox virus and the less pathogenic cowpox virus. This was not a route to developing vaccines that was available for other diseases.

The next major leap was the concept of attenuation developed by Louis Pasteur in the 19th century, which we heard about in Chapter 3. Pasteur's discovery is the basis for the viral vaccines we currently use against measles, mumps, rubella, polio (the OPV form), chickenpox, rotavirus and tuberculosis.

It would take the best part of a century for Louis Pasteur's brilliance to come to full fruition. The golden age of immunisation and widespread control of major infectious diseases did not start until the mid-20th century. Throughout the 19th century, however, scientists made vital progress in growing and understanding the bacteria that can cause devastating human diseases. This was essential groundwork that enabled the later development of vaccines. German microbiologists played an important role, although scientists in France and Italy also made significant contributions.

In this chapter, I will consider the extraordinary progress we have made in developing vaccines to help keep our children healthy throughout life.

Tetanus

Edwin Smith was an enigma. Born in Orlando, Florida, he became a scholar, specialising in Egyptian antiquities, but was not averse to dabbling in a bit of antiques forgery. In 1862, while in Luxor, he bought a papyrus from a dealer called Mustapha Aga. The papyrus was long but in poor condition, and was written in a script Smith could not read. He kept the papyrus until he died, when his daughter gave it to the New York Historical Society, which had it translated in 1930. The translation showed that it was a medical text – but one completely unlike the few other surviving Egyptian medical texts, which are based on magic.

The Edwin Smith Papyrus, as it is now called, is the oldest known treatise on surgery and may have been a military surgical manual. It describes 48 patients – probably all soldiers – in remarkable clinical detail, using an almost contemporary scientific approach. It dates to 1600 BC, but the writing is hurried and contains multiple errors. Experts believe it is plagiarised from an even older papyrus attributed to the great Egyptian physician Imhotep, who lived 1000 years earlier.

The papyrus includes the first known description of tetanus (the terms *tepau* and *metu* have no modern equivalents):

> If you find in that patient that his flesh has developed
> heat under the wound which is in the *tepau* of his skull.
> That man, he has developed toothache under the site of
> that injury. You put your hand on him and you find his
> brow is wet with sweat. The muscles (*metu*) of his neck
> are taut, his face is flushed, his teeth and his back. The
> odour inside his braincase is like sheep/goat excrement. His
> mouth is bound, his eyebrows drawn, his face as if he was
> weeping.

The toothache resulting from the soldier's clenched jaw was due to tetanus, also known as 'lockjaw'. His facial expression was the sardonic grimace or smile known as the *risus sardonicus*; tetanus was also called 'the grinning death'. Hippocrates recognised the clinical features of agonising muscle spasms in the war-wounded 1000 years after the Egyptians, and named the disease *tetanos*, meaning 'muscular spasm'.

Tetanus is a truly frightening disease, characterised by muscle rigidity and convulsive spasms. The muscle stiffness often involves the jaw and neck and then becomes generalised. At its worst, patients with spasms of the spine will arch themselves into a position called opisthotonus.

Physicians may have known millennia ago of the link between tetanus and war wounds, but it is only a little over a century since scientists showed that the cause of tetanus in fact lies in the very ground on which we walk, and in the soil where our wounded fell.

In the late 1880s, a German Jewish doctor, Arthur Nicolaier, isolated a toxin from soil with similar properties to strychnine, which would later be shown to be tetanus toxin. The tetanus vaccine we have used for almost a century is a toxoid made by treating tetanus toxin with formaldehyde (similar to the diphtheria toxoid).

Nicolaier was a highly influential physician. He was appointed as Professor of Medicine in Berlin in 1921, but was removed from his post by the Nazis in 1933, and committed suicide in 1942 when about to be sent to Theresienstadt concentration camp. How tragic that a man whose work led to the development of a tetanus toxoid vaccine that protected World War II troops against a horrible, painful death should lose his own life at the hands of the Nazis.

The link between tetanus and war is a poignant one. The disease is caused by a nerve toxin produced by the bacterium *Clostridium tetani*, which grows in the gut of cattle and horses, so it is widely distributed in the soil in farming areas. Hence a field of war is a breeding ground for tetanus, particularly if the field has been manured.

The warfare creates the wounds that allow the tetanus organism to enter the body and set up an infection, which in turn generates the tetanus toxin that attacks the nerves.

World War I saw widespread tetanus in all its horror. A century before, a muzzle-loading musket could fire four shots a minute to a distance of less than 100 metres. By the early 20th century, machine guns could fire hundreds of rounds a minute over several thousand metres. The war wounds these guns inflicted were often contaminated by soil in the heavily fertilised fields of Flanders and northern France. A third of all British soldiers wounded in 1914 were racked by the muscle spasms of tetanus within days. More than half of all the soldiers who developed tetanus in World War I died.

A French veterinarian, Edmond Nocard, had shown in 1897 that tetanus antitoxin could treat tetanus or prevent it in the war-wounded. After the initial catastrophic mortality in the early months of World War I, soldiers with contaminated wounds were given prophylactic injections of anti-tetanus horse serum. This preventative treatment dramatically reduced the incidence of tetanus on both sides of the conflict. There were occasional deaths from anaphylactic reaction to the horse serum, but historians estimate that the use of antitoxin after those first disastrous months saved the lives of as many as half a million wounded soldiers.

In the early 1920s, another French veterinarian, Gaston Ramon, developed a method for treating tetanus toxin with formaldehyde to make it less potent, leading in 1924 to the development of tetanus toxoid vaccine by his colleague Pierre Descombey. This is the tetanus toxoid vaccine we still use for routine immunisations in childhood. We also use a 'booster' dose of tetanus toxoid vaccine to increase immunity in a child or adult who suffers a tetanus-prone injury, such as a deep cut sustained on a sports field, or a battlefield wound contaminated with soil.

Tetanus toxoid vaccine was of major importance and used by virtually all countries in World War II. Only a handful of individuals died from tetanus throughout the entire war.

An important aspect of tetanus immunisation is that tetanus is acquired through a contaminated wound, and is not passed from person to person – a person with tetanus cannot infect another person. A child who has not received any childhood immunisations is not protected against tetanus, no matter how many other children have been immunised.

I have seen tetanus in African newborns who caught it from their mothers at birth because their cut umbilical stump was traditionally packed with mud. The newborns were rigid, and if someone made a loud sound, such as shutting a door noisily, they all started to spasm at once. Almost all such newborns die. (I'll talk about this more in Chapter 9, on vaccines and pregnancy.)

I have seen it in a few older unimmunised children. A seven-year-old girl whom I helped treat in Oxford was admitted to hospital with what was first thought to be epilepsy. A physician who had seen tetanus in Africa witnessed the girl go into an arching spasm when the door banged and correctly diagnosed tetanus. She had caught it when her parents had her ears pierced in an Oxfordshire marketplace. Her spasms were excruciatingly painful, but at least she survived. Not all children do.

Geriatricians see tetanus in elderly men and women who were never immunised and are infected when gardening; the recipe is a simple prick from a rose-thorn and just a whiff of manure. An unimmunised child or adult who cuts their foot on a rusty nail is also at risk (as we will hear in Chapter 13).

Whooping cough

Whooping cough, or pertussis, has been recognised since the Middle Ages. The term whooping cough, which was sometimes written as 'hooping cough', was first recorded in England in 1190. The word 'pertussis' is Latin for 'forceful cough', and the 'whoop' of whooping cough describes the characteristic intake of breath (inward gasp) at the end of each bout of coughing. Another name was 'chin-cough'. The Scots called it 'the kink', meaning a fit or paroxysm. The bouts, or paroxysms, of uncontrollable coughing may end in convulsions (fits).

Although they could describe the disease well, pre-20th century physicians had some strange ideas on how to treat it. Nicholas Culpeper, a 17th-century herbalist, suggested that rosemary should be 'taken in a pipe, as tobacco is taken' by both adults and children suffering from whooping cough. Purgatives and emetics were often prescribed, and the use of diuretics and bleeding by leeches were also commonplace. In 1726, a Dr Willis recommended giving a child with whooping cough a 'sudden fright'. He also used 'cupping', an ancient, painful and ineffective remedy that involves applying cups emptied of air to the body, thereby creating suction and raising welts or blisters. Dr Willis favoured cupping round the neck, behind the ears and under the armpits. Around the same time there was a fashion for treating children with infusions containing hemlock, which is a bit of a 'kill or cure' approach – hemlock was the poison the ancient Greek philosopher Socrates famously drank to carry out his own death sentence.

In 1898, one doctor reported:

There are many curious customs and superstitions existing even in this enlightened age, and among the most peculiar are some practised by the peasants of Ireland for the cure of various complaints. In certain districts of that country whooping cough is treated in quite a unique manner. A few months ago much amusement was caused by a case

which came before the Coroner's Court in Belfast, in which
whooping cough was treated in a child by passing the
sufferer three times under a donkey ... Some donkeys are
believed to be possessed of curative virtues in a much higher
degree than are others. A man living in County Cork owned
an animal which could boast of more than a local reputation.
This man used to lead his donkey through the streets of the
City of Cork, crying out: 'Will any one come under my ass
for the chin-cough?'

Whooping cough classically causes epidemics every three to four
years. During an epidemic most susceptible children are infected
before the disease burns itself out. As new children are born,
the number of susceptible children mounts gradually until there
are enough for the next epidemic to occur. Primary-school-age
children are most commonly affected, but people of any age can
catch pertussis, from newborn to elderly.

It often goes unrecognised in adults. I remember seeing a
dentist friend doubled over in an uncontrollable bout of coughing.

'How long have you had that cough?' I asked suspiciously.

'Three weeks.'

'Have your children been coughing too?'

'Yes, for a month.'

'I think you've got whooping cough.'

'Thank goodness. I can't breathe and I thought I was dying.'

Adults don't die from pertussis, but what the Chinese
accurately call the 100-day cough can be so troublesome they
sometimes wish they could. Infants younger than three months
can die from the condition. Older infants and children get
uncontrollable bouts of coughing that cause them to go blue

in the face and often vomit. The coughing keeps the child and the whole family awake at night for weeks, until everyone is completely exhausted.

The organism that causes whooping cough was first grown in 1906 by Belgians Jules Bordet and Octave Gengou. It was given the name *Bordetella pertussis*, which honours Bordet, but they both got their names on the medium they developed for growing the organism, Bordet-Gengou medium. Unusually, it contains potato. I can't help wondering if one of them accidentally spilt their lunch onto the tissue-culture plate and found it was the ideal culture medium.

Whole-cell vaccines made from inactivated pertussis in culture started to be developed just before World War I. The whole-cell vaccine got its name because whole killed cells of *Bordetella pertussis* were used to make the vaccine. The so-called acellular pertussis vaccines used in most industrialised countries nowadays are made from a small number of the organism's proteins, not the whole organism. The first licensed pertussis vaccine was made by an American paediatrician, Leila Denmark, in the early 1930s. She was just the third woman ever to graduate in medicine from the University of Georgia, and was quite a character. She was ahead of her time in saying that pregnant women should not take certain medicines, adults should not smoke around children, and too much sugar was harmful – even on her 100th birthday, she refused to eat cake. All of this seemed to work, as she lived to the venerable age of 114.

Pertussis vaccination programs were started in Australia in 1942. Australia introduced the DTP (diphtheria-tetanus-pertussis) triple vaccine in 1953, both in the routine infant immunisation program and in schools.

Meningitis

The moon carries the masks of meningitis into bedrooms,
fills the wombs of pregnant women with cold water and,
as soon as I'm not careful, throws handfuls of grass on my
shoulders.

The Public, Federico García Lorca (1898–1936)

What remained was a pale, prematurely aged face, a
gruesome mask with simplified features, in which nothing
could be read but pain and disgust and profound horror.

Rosshalde, Hermann Hesse (1877–1962)

In his short novel *Rosshalde,* Hermann Hesse describes the death
of young Pierre from meningitis. But doctors my age do not need
to read classic literature to know about meningitis.

When I was a young doctor, bacterial meningitis was a
common and much-feared disease in infants and preschool-age
children, and the hospital where I work would look after 20
to 25 children with meningitis every year. The children would
frequently develop fever, a bulging fontanelle and a stiff neck, and
would often have convulsions or just look ill and unresponsive.
Feeling helpless, their parents would watch aghast what was
happening to their beloved child.

Nowadays, although our hospital admits more children
than ever before, we may not see a single child with bacterial
meningitis all year. The difference is immunisation.

The commonest cause of meningitis by far is an organism called
Haemophilus influenzae type b (Hib for short). Before a vaccine

was developed, some 5 to 10% of children with Hib meningitis would die and about 20% would be left with permanent brain damage, which could result in cerebral palsy, epilepsy, deafness, blindness and intellectual impairment. Hib can also cause a life-threatening illness called epiglottitis, a severe swelling of the top of the windpipe, which can cause a child to suffocate, as with diphtheria. Children can also get other nasty infections from Hib, including pneumonia, osteomyelitis and septic arthritis (acute infections of the bone and joints, respectively).

Before immunisation began in the 1990s, over 500 children under five years old in Australia developed severe Hib infections each year. Aboriginal children were particularly susceptible. In the United States, 20,000 children per year had Hib infections, a high proportion of them indigenous children. The reasons indigenous children worldwide are at increased risk are unclear, though the causes are probably mainly environmental, such as closer family contact and factors related to social disadvantage.

Following the introduction of vaccines in both countries, Hib disease is now vanishingly rare. Australia introduced Hib vaccines into the routine schedule in 1993, and within a short time there was a 95% decrease in incidence. Most of our young doctors have never seen a child with Hib meningitis, and I have not seen one for more than 20 years.

Incidentally, Hib incidence in Australia fell much more quickly than expected, to the extent that even unimmunised children are now less likely to get Hib infection. This is an example of vaccine-induced herd immunity (which we looked at in Chapter 1). It happens with Hib vaccine because the vaccine gets rid of Hib from immunised children's noses, and the main way Hib is transmitted between children is through their nasal secretions.

Hib immunisation is not yet available universally, and much of the world is not so lucky: in 2000, experts estimate over 8 million children developed Hib infection worldwide and 370,000 of them died. However, by 2016, global efforts to bring Hib vaccine to the developing world had ensured that 191 countries had Hib vaccine in their routine childhood immunisation schedules. Global coverage of Hib vaccine was 70%, but with considerable inequity: the coverage was 90% in the Americas but only 28% in the Western Pacific. However, considerable recent progress has been made in Southeast Asia, where the proportion of children immunised against Hib rose from 56% in 2015 to 80% in 2016. At this rate it may be possible to eradicate Hib disease from the world.

The other major causes of bacterial meningitis in infants and young children are organisms called *Streptococcus pneumoniae* (pneumococcus for short) and *Neisseria meningitidis* (meningococcus). Although as the name suggests the main disease caused by pneumococcus is pneumonia, when it causes meningitis it is actually the most devastating of the three organisms. The mortality is higher and children who recover are more likely to be left with brain damage.

Immunisation against pneumococci with the best vaccines available, so-called conjugate pneumococcal vaccines, was introduced into the routine Australian childhood schedule in 2001 and has been highly effective. Conjugate pneumococcal vaccines are increasingly being introduced into developing countries through philanthropic funding of vaccine programs. Pneumococcal immunisation provides another example of vaccine-induced herd immunity: when the conjugate vaccine is introduced routinely in infancy, the incidence of pneumococcal disease also falls in the unimmunised population.

Meningococcal meningitis has a lower mortality than Hib or pneumococcal meningitis, but sometimes you can die or be maimed for life from meningococcal bloodstream infection before you have the chance to develop meningitis.

Marty Mayfield was a teenager who lived for skiing. He dreamed of being selected for the Australian Olympic Team. Every holiday he would train with an elite squad. At age 17, when he was at a ski training camp, he began to feel exhausted and ached all over. He was sure he had the flu. But in a matter of hours a rash appeared on his legs and he was rushed to hospital and went into a coma. In his dreams he had lost his legs and was floating in the sky.

When he woke from the coma, his father was sitting by the bed. He was fighting back emotion and trying to tell Marty something.

'I know, Dad. I've lost my legs, haven't I?'

Marty was determined to become a medical student to prevent this from happening to others. He was equally determined to ski again.

I met Marty when, as a medical student, he applied to do a research project with me on fever and rash. 'I'm particularly interested in this topic because I had meningococcal infection myself,' he told me as he sat in my room.

'At least it didn't have any lasting effects on you,' I said.

'Except for my legs,' he replied casually, and lifted his trouser bottoms to show me two artificial legs. Marty had just returned from Vancouver, where he had won the silver medal in downhill skiing at the Paralympics.

Meningococcal infection can occur in outbreaks. It can hit teenagers and university students, unlike Hib and pneumococcal meningitis, which are diseases of pre-school children. It can kill or maim within hours. As such, meningococcal infections tend to get more publicity than Hib or pneumococcal infections, but we now have vaccines against all three. They are not perfect and they do not yet prevent every case, but they certainly prevent the vast majority.

All the organisms that cause childhood meningitis, Hib, pneumococcus and meningococcus, get in through the victim's nose. Often they just stay happily inside the nose, lazing in a warm bath of mucus, reproducing intermittently, and doing the host no harm whatsoever. All right for some. But if the organism moves to the nose of a new host who has never experienced it before, it can sometimes pass through the nose lining (nasal mucosa) and get into the blood vessels to cause bloodstream infection (septicaemia, which in the case of meningococcus is called meningococcaemia).

Meningococcal septicaemia can clot up big blood vessels, causing loss of large areas of skin and underlying tissue, which will need skin grafts if the child recovers. At its worst the child can lose limbs, sometimes all four. As with Marty, the infection can be so rampant that a child, young adult or older person can go from well to moribund in a matter of hours. Sometimes it is so fulminant (severe) that even immediate diagnosis and treatment with penicillin, the most effective antibiotic, cannot save the person's life. Meningococcal infection is one of the most feared of all infections.

Pneumonia

The lung infection pneumonia was described by the ancient physician Hippocrates, but he called it a disease 'named by the ancients', so it had clearly been around long before the fifth century BC. In the 12th century, the medieval Jewish philosopher and physician Maimonides wrote: 'The basic symptoms that occur in pneumonia and that are never lacking are as follows: acute fever, sticking pleuritic pain in the side, short rapid breaths, serrated pulse and cough.' The pleura is the membrane surrounding the lung, and when it becomes inflamed, as can happen with pneumonia, it hurts a lot to cough or take a deep breath, a condition called pleurisy.

Before the advent of antibiotics to treat pneumonia it had a high mortality rate, and in 1918 the legendary Canadian physician Sir William Osler described it as the 'captain of the men of death'. Even now, pneumonia is a major cause of child hospitalisation throughout the world, and kills over a million children a year, 95% of them in developing countries.

Pneumococcus (*Streptococcus pneumoniae*), one of the causes of meningitis, is the major cause of bacterial pneumonia. Susceptibility depends on age, with the highest rates in infancy and again in old age, as immunity wanes. The other major risk factor is tobacco smoke, either through smoking or through living with a smoker. Aboriginal people are at particularly high risk of pneumococcal infection throughout their lives, partly due to tobacco smoke exposure and other associations with disadvantage. We have had effective vaccines against pneumococcus only since the year 2000, but they are now included in the routine childhood schedule in all industrialised countries and increasing numbers of developing countries.

In infancy, pneumonia is usually caused by a virus called respiratory syncytial virus (RSV); despite many years of effort by some of our best scientists, we have not been able to develop an effective vaccine against it. RSV was first isolated from

134

chimpanzees with colds in 1956 and from human infants a year later.

A killed RSV vaccine was used in limited trials in the United States in the late 1960s. Disastrously, children given the killed RSV vaccine actually got worse-than-usual infections when they caught RSV. Two died. The trial was hastily stopped before any further children were immunised. That tragedy has led to extra caution, and is one of the reasons we have no RSV vaccine, even though RSV is a disease of global significance. (More on that in Chapter 15.)

Influenza is a major cause of pneumonia at all ages, although the mortality increases with age (as will be discussed in Chapter 10). We have vaccines against influenza, but because the influenza virus mutates ('changes its spots') annually, we need a new dose of influenza vaccine every year.

Tuberculosis is also a major cause of pneumonia globally, but predominantly in developing countries (as discussed in Chapter 5).

Hepatitis

Hepatitis means 'inflammation of the liver'. It can be caused by infections, usually viruses, and sometimes by other things such as medications, autoimmune diseases and allergies. Acute hepatitis can result in a debilitating illness involving jaundice, vomiting and anorexia.

The major viruses that cause hepatitis are inventively named hepatitis A, hepatitis B and hepatitis C. We have extremely safe and highly effective vaccines against two of these – the hepatitis B vaccine was first approved in 1981 and the hepatitis A vaccine was introduced in the early 1990s. As yet there is no vaccine for hepatitis C, although vaccines are being developed and we do have new, safer oral antiviral drugs to treat the disease.

Hepatitis A is also called infectious hepatitis, and is caught by eating or drinking contaminated food ('contaminated' is a euphemistic way of saying that the virus is shed in a person's faeces and spread to food). Doctors say that transmission occurs by the faecal–oral route. That is why, when it comes to food, people visiting countries with a high prevalence of hepatitis A should 'wash it, peel it, cook it or forget it'. But travellers can be more certain of avoiding hepatitis A by getting themselves immunised with hepatitis A vaccine, or the combined hepatitis A and B vaccine.

Hepatitis B virus is also called serum hepatitis, and is acquired from injecting blood or blood products contaminated with hepatitis B virus. The virus is extremely infectious and can be passed on by contact with very small amounts of virus. It is 50 to 100 times more infectious than HIV.

Most people know that intravenous drug users are at risk of catching hepatitis B because of needle-sharing, and many look askance at *anyone* with chronic (long-term) hepatitis B virus infection. Hepatitis B can also be passed on in blood transfusions and contaminated blood products; in the past, before we knew the cause and how to prevent it, men with haemophilia used to catch hepatitis B from their treatment with the blood-clotting protein Factor VIII.

People with chronic hepatitis B can pass hepatitis B to their partners during sexual intercourse. In 1967, Swedish doctors reported an outbreak of 568 cases of hepatitis B infection among Swedish cross-country runners, occurring over the years 1957 to 1963. The tentative explanation was that all the runners had suffered scratches and skin lacerations, and the virus had been caught from small drops of blood on bushes, or from shared water when the runners washed together after running. Of course, it is possible that many of the runners had sex with each other, but history does not relate whether that alternative theory was even considered. Whatever the cause, there was a lot of hepatitis B transmitted between runners. (These were the days before hepatitis B immunisation was available.)

Hepatitis B can also be transmitted in contact sports. In 1982 in Japan, half of the 10 members of a high-school sumo wrestling club developed hepatitis B in one year, transmitted by a club member who was unaware he had chronic hepatitis B infection. Wrestlers in the club were known to keep wrestling even when they were injured and bleeding from skin wounds.

As recently as 2000, 11 of 65 members of a United States university football team developed hepatitis B infection. Five became acutely ill with hepatitis and six remained asymptomatic. Again, the source was a player with chronic hepatitis B infection.

The football team outbreak illustrates an important point. If an unimmunised child or adult catches hepatitis B infection, they may develop acute hepatitis (acute inflammation of the liver, causing an enlarged, tender liver and yellow jaundice), which can sometimes be fatal, or they may have a 'sub-clinical' infection, meaning they become infected but have no symptoms. You are much more likely to catch hepatitis B from an infected person who is perfectly well than from someone who is bright yellow. Nowadays, though, none of the athletes just described would have been infected, because they would have been immunised at birth or at school.

Most people with acute (short-term) hepatitis B recover after weeks of being unwell, and remain immune, but some will die rapidly from liver failure. A few will develop chronic hepatitis B infection, although the commonest way of developing this is at birth, if you are unfortunate enough to have a mother with chronic hepatitis B. People with chronic hepatitis B infection are often perfectly well for years, but the virus is living in their liver and in their bloodstream, and can eventually damage the liver. Chronic inflammation of the liver can lead to cirrhosis or to liver cancer. Liver cirrhosis causes massive build-up of fluid in the abdomen (ascites) and can lead to blood vomits (haematemesis) and early death. I will discuss how hepatitis B immunisation prevents liver cancer in Chapter 8.

Gastroenteritis

Rotavirus is the most virulent cause of gastroenteritis (gastro). There is a strong Australian connection here, because rotavirus was first identified in 1973 by an Australian team, including Ruth Bishop, a virologist, and Graeme Barnes, a gastroenterologist. They detected viruses in the intestinal cells of children with gastroenteritis. Initially they called them 'duoviruses' because they came from the duodenum. Later the viruses were renamed 'rotaviruses' because of their wheel-like structure (*rota* is Latin for 'wheel'). This was a vital step on the road to developing a rotavirus vaccine.

Rotavirus is a virus that almost all infants catch. It infects the gastrointestinal tract (gut) and causes vomiting, profuse watery diarrhoea, abdominal pain and fever. Infants and young children are most likely to become ill, although older children and adults can also catch rotavirus. The most severely affected infants have to be admitted to hospital for rehydration, often using a drip to give intravenous fluids.

For a long time gastroenteritis was the major killer of young children worldwide, leading to the deaths of some 5 million infants and toddlers a year, and rotavirus is still a big killer of children in developing countries. In 2013, an estimated 215,000 children under five died from rotavirus gastroenteritis, 195,000 in developing countries and 20,000 in industrialised countries.

For a long time the WHO focused on improved treatment using oral rehydration solutions containing sugar, salt and water. However, deaths due to rotavirus infection continued to occur. Rotavirus vaccines were developed as live attenuated vaccines that are given orally, so that the vaccine virus can stimulate an immune response in the gut. They have led to a marked drop in diarrhoeal diseases and in hospitalisations for rotavirus.

There were one or two deaths from rotavirus each year in Australia before the introduction of rotavirus vaccine in 2006, and half of those were Aboriginal children. In the United States there were 20 to 60 deaths each year, and Native American and Alaskan Native children were at higher risk. This may have been due to close living conditions, but essentially rotavirus gastroenteritis is a disease of poverty. Social disadvantage increases susceptibility to infection – a persisting gap between rich and poor that needs to be addressed. Immunisation is a powerful way of narrowing that gap.

By 2016, rotavirus vaccine had been introduced into 90 countries, of which 68 had achieved over 50% infant coverage. The WHO estimated rotavirus vaccine global coverage at 25% in 2016.

We will hear more about rotavirus in Chapter 11.

Measles

Measles will always show you if someone isn't doing a
good job on vaccinations. Kids will start dying of
measles.

Bill Gates, founder of Microsoft (born 1955)

Few adults nowadays and almost none of our junior doctors
have seen measles. Most children with measles are very miserable
but recover, and people sometimes play down the severity of the
disease and the need for the vaccine. But at its worst, measles
was and still is a fearsome disease. A ninth-century Iranian
physician, Muhammad ibn Zakariya al-Razi, was the first person
to distinguish measles from smallpox.

Although smallpox came to Australia with the First Fleet in
1788 and decimated the local Aboriginal population within a
year, measles did not come with the First Fleet. An Australian
epidemiology research student, Beverley Paterson, determined
to discover when measles first arrived in Australia, took on the
arduous and inventive step of searching the logbooks of ship
surgeons on voyages from England to Australia between 1829
and 1882. She also examined quarantine records. She found that
no ship passengers were quarantined with measles before 1850,
but ships arriving after that had many passengers who needed
quarantining because of measles.

The surgeons' logbooks showed the reason. Before 1850,
ship voyages from England to Australia took about six months.
If measles broke out, the only people safe from infection were
those who had had measles before. Otherwise measles spread like
wildfire, killing 1 in 10 infected. By the time the ships reached

Australia everyone was either dead or immune, and there was no measles virus left to transmit.

The year 1850 was the very year that faster and larger American clippers started plying the voyage from England to Australia. They almost halved the time of the journey, which meant that some people were still infectious with measles when the ships arrived. Other factors in spreading measles to Australia were the removal of restrictions on the number of children permitted on ships and the huge influx of immigrants trying to get rich during the Gold Rush.

One dose of measles vaccine or a vaccine such as measles-mumps-rubella (MMR) vaccine protects at least 95% of those vaccinated against clinical measles. Measles vaccine was licensed in the United States in 1963 and the number of measles cases and measles deaths plummeted within four years. Over 35 million cases of measles are estimated to have been prevented in the United States since then. Measles vaccine was registered in Australia in 1968 and routine childhood immunisation started in 1970 in all States and Territories except New South Wales, where it started in 1972.

MMR vaccine is given at an age when children often catch virus infections in daycare or from older siblings. If a child develops new symptoms soon after receiving MMR vaccine, these symptoms may be caused by the vaccine (true adverse effect) or may be due to a different virus infection (coincidental).

A 1986 study in Finland neatly teased out this issue. The authors recruited 581 pairs of twins due to receive MMR vaccine and gave one twin of each pair the vaccine and the other twin a placebo injection in a randomised double-blind controlled trial. (We heard about these in Chapter 5.) Three weeks later, the twins received the other injection, so that each child ended up receiving one dose of MMR and one of inactive placebo.

The researchers then compared the children's symptoms following MMR vaccine with those following the placebo. Children given the placebo had as many episodes of diarrhoea and vomiting and as many episodes of coughing and wheezing as children given MMR vaccine, showing that these symptoms were likely to be coincidence; the child was going to show them anyway. MMR vaccine was found to be significantly more likely than placebo to cause fever and rash about a week after the injection, so it was a true adverse effect due to a mild case of measles.

In 1980, before the measles vaccine was widely available, an estimated 2.6 million children died in the world each year from measles. Although that number has fallen by about 95% since then, it means that, based on WHO estimates, 134,200 children died from measles in 2015, or 367 children every day – an unacceptably high number.

Measles can still, in this day and age, kill or maim a child in any country in the world. But numbers alone do not do justice to the horror of the disease. I have seen previously healthy, chubby children whose brains were destroyed by measles encephalitis, the disease that killed Roald Dahl's daughter Olivia. If they survived, they could not speak or walk. I have seen children so badly infected by measles pneumonia that they had to be artificially paralysed and put on a ventilator in our intensive care unit.

In Africa, measles is a major killer. Children who are not already malnourished when they catch the disease are more susceptible to diarrhoeal illnesses and are at risk of dying for up to a year after they recover from measles. In 1974, I did my medical student elective in Moshi in Tanzania, at the foot of

Mount Kilimanjaro. In the mission hospital there, I saw wards of children dying from measles pneumonia despite the antibiotics we gave them. Sometimes measles ate away their cheeks, a condition called 'noma'. I saw an attractive young girl brought into the hospital with half her head wrapped in a shawl. When I removed the shawl, there was a gaping hole in her cheek through which I could see her teeth and tongue.

There is only one strain of measles and no animal population harbouring the disease, which means it should be possible to get rid of measles altogether through immunisation. The WHO hopes to eradicate measles from five global regions by 2020, and eventually from the entire world. The reason we have not succeeded in doing so already is that measles is much more infectious than smallpox and spreads more readily and more rapidly.

Because of this high infectiousness, at least 93% of children need to be immunised to achieve herd immunity and prevent measles from circulating in a community. When this high level is achieved, as it has been in most parts of the United States and Australia, measles no longer circulates. However, 1 in 20 immunised children is still susceptible to infection. Thus if measles is introduced by someone from overseas it can start to circulate again. If it gets into an unimmunised or poorly immunised section of the population, such as those with cultural or religious objections, it can cause a large outbreak that will infect almost all unimmunised children and 1 in 20 immunised children.

A 2014 outbreak in Ohio infected 383 people, of whom 340 were unimmunised. Virtually all of the measles cases (99%) were among the Amish community, which has a religious objection to vaccination. Herd immunity prevented measles from spreading more extensively among the rest of the highly immunised community.

We want measles to disappear completely, like smallpox, and we may eventually succeed in making that happen. But at present, and for the foreseeable future, measles is more like diphtheria: if we let our guard down and stop immunising, it will return with a vengeance.

Mumps

The old English word 'mump' means to mope. I don't know if you're getting bored with hearing this, but Hippocrates recognised mumps about 2500 years ago. (It's not hard to see why Hippocrates is held in such high esteem by contemporary doctors worldwide. He was a brilliant clinician, and one who thought profoundly about ethics; he also communicated well, leaving us his thoughts in writing in perpetuity.) Hippocrates described the clinical features of mumps in the first book of his work, *Epidemics*, and clearly explained how mumps can be complicated by orchitis (testicular inflammation):

> Swellings appeared about the ears, in many on either side, and in the greatest number on both sides, being unaccompanied by fever so as to confine the patient to bed; in all cases they disappeared without giving trouble, neither did any of them come to suppuration [develop pus], as is common in swellings from other causes. They were of a lax, large, diffused character, without inflammation or pain, and they went away without any critical sign. They seized children, adults, and mostly those who were engaged in the exercises of the *palestra* [wrestling school] and gymnasium, but seldom attacked women. Many had dry coughs without

expectoration, and accompanied with hoarseness of voice. In some instances earlier, and in others later, inflammations with pain seized sometimes one of the testicles, and sometimes both; some of these were accompanied with fever and some not; the greater part of these were attended with much suffering. In other respects they were free of disease, so as not to require medical assistance.

We now know mumps is caused by a virus with a predilection for the salivary glands, particularly the parotid gland (the largest of the salivary glands). Mumps parotitis, meaning inflammation of the parotid gland, results in a miserable child with a sore, swollen neck for a few days. But mumps virus can also cause meningitis and mumps meningitis used to be the commonest form of childhood meningitis. It has a much better prognosis than bacterial meningitis or measles encephalitis, but it still leads to headache, vomiting and a hospital admission.

Other complications of mumps are the extraordinarily painful pancreatitis (inflammation of the pancreas), orchitis (painful swelling of the testicles) in boys and young men as described by Hippocrates, and oophoritis (swelling of the ovary or ovaries, causing severe abdominal pain) in girls and young women. Orchitis can sometimes cause testicular atrophy (small testes) and sterility.

You might hope parents would be more worried about their children's brains than their genitalia. However, when the MMR vaccine was introduced into the United Kingdom in 1988, the biggest selling point was not preventing measles encephalitis or congenital rubella or mumps meningitis, but preventing male sterility. What a surprise.

Mumps vaccines were introduced in Australia in 1980 and a combined measles and mumps vaccine was used from 1982 until 1989, when it was supplanted by measles-mumps-rubella (MMR) vaccine. The measles, mumps and rubella components of the vaccine are made by growing and then attenuating each virus; it is a live attenuated vaccine.

Rubella

Rubella is sometimes called German measles, because German physicians were the first to describe it as a separate condition from measeles and scarlet fever, which it resembled. The first clinical description of rubella was Friedrich Hoffmann's in 1740; two other Germans, de Bergen and Orlow (their first names seem to have been lost to posterity), confirmed these clinical findings in the 1750s. Yet another German, George de Maton, suggested in 1814 that rubella was indeed different from measles and scarlet fever. An English Royal Artillery surgeon, Henry Veale, first used the name 'rubella' (Latin for 'reddish') when describing an outbreak in India in 1866.

Rubella is a mild disease, with a faint rash and few complications, except occasionally a transient arthritis. The peak age range for catching it is five to nine years old. But the main reason for rubella immunisation is to prevent pregnant women from catching the disease and giving birth to infants with congenital rubella syndrome. (I will discuss rubella in detail in Chapter 9, on vaccines in pregnancy.)

Before immunisation, most girls used to catch rubella in childhood, but a small number were still susceptible as they entered child-bearing age. Australia started rubella immunisation of

12- to 14-year-old schoolgirls as a school-based program in 1971. But because boys were not immunised, rubella still circulated. This meant girls who missed out on the school program, and girls or young women who emigrated from Southeast Asia, where rubella does not circulate so much, were often non-immune and susceptible to the disease in pregnancy.

In 1989 Australia introduced measles-mumps-rubella (MMR) vaccine for all boys and girls at 12 months of age. As in the United States, Australian children are given a second dose at 18 months, to improve measles immunity. Rubella no longer circulates and congenital rubella has now virtually disappeared in Australia: there were only five children born with congenital rubella syndrome between 2001 and 2013, and all were to mothers born overseas who had not received rubella vaccine.

Varicella

The same virus, varicella zoster virus (VZV), causes both chickenpox and zoster (shingles). This is because after a child develops chickenpox, the virus can remain latent in the sensory nerves for years without causing any symptoms. But in times of stress or when the immune system is impaired, the chickenpox virus can re-emerge as shingles.

VZV is a herpesvirus and these features of latency and reactivation are common to all herpesviruses (the Greek word *herpein* means 'to creep'). For example, herpes simplex virus causes a severe mouth infection in infants with ulcers of the mouth and throat. Cold sores are a reactivation of the herpes simplex virus, which has been lying latent in the nerves of the lips. Almost everyone catches herpes simplex when young, but not everyone gets cold sores. Almost everyone catches chickenpox when young, but not everyone gets shingles.

When I am feeling wicked, I ask my medical students: 'What is the difference between herpesviruses and true love?' The answer is that herpesviruses are forever.

Like me, you may be relieved to know that Hippocrates did not describe chickenpox – it is nice to know he was human after all. But the ancient Greeks have given us the name 'zoster', first used in the 19th century and taken from their word for a girdle. The word 'shingles' was first used in the 18th century and comes from the Latin *cingulus* (belt). Both refer to the most common manifestation of shingles, which is in a belt-like distribution on one side of the body, around the lower abdomen.

Nobody knows how chickenpox got its strange name. One theory is that an Old English word *giccan*, meaning 'to itch', was corrupted into 'chicken'. In 1730, English physician Thomas Fuller published a book on rashes called *Exanthemologia* in which he suggested the name derived from 'the smallness of the Specks, which our Women might fancy looked as tho' a Child had been picked with the Bills of Chickens'. The English writer Samuel Johnson was unconvinced, and in his famous 1755 *Dictionary of the English Language*, he wrote that chickenpox got its name 'from its being of no very great danger'.

Over a century later, Charles Fagge wrote in his book *The Principles and Practice of Medicine* (published in 1886) that the fluid-filled vesicles looked like chickpeas. Another theory is that chicken was a word for a little child and it is mostly children who catch chickenpox. Chickenpox is notoriously itchy, and the name could also be a corruption of the term 'itching-pox'.

Jeff Aronson, an Oxford pharmacologist and wordsmith, gives his own explanation. In Shakespeare's time there was an English gold coin called a chequeen; Shakespeare features it in his play *Pericles, Prince of Tyre*. The chequeen was used as currency in 15th-century India, where the name was often corrupted to 'chickeen' or 'chick'. It was worth about four rupees; in other words, not very much. Aronson conjectures that this word gave rise to the name 'chickenpox' because chickenpox was seen as an insignificant, or cheap, infection (no pun intended) compared with smallpox.

It is rather wonderful that we will never know which of these inventive suggestions is correct, but we do know chickens have nothing material to do with chickenpox.

As noted earlier, in the 18th century physicians thought wrongly that chickenpox was a mild form of smallpox. (Varicella, another name for chickenpox, means 'little smallpox'.) Just as wrong-headed were some of the methods used to treat it. In County Down in Ireland during the 19th century, remedies for chickenpox included 'two kinds of food obtained from two first cousins who are married, and soup made from the tails of mice'.

In fact, although they both cause pocks, smallpox and chickenpox are caused by very different viruses. It was not until 1888 that a German physician, Janus von Bokay, reported a number of cases of children who developed chickenpox two weeks after being in contact with someone with zoster, suggesting they had caught chickenpox from that person and that chickenpox and zoster were caused by the same virus.

Chickenpox or varicella is usually a fairly mild if annoying illness. A young child is covered in very itchy spots, mainly on the trunk and face. They may also be in the throat or on the eyelids, which can make the child miserable. The skin sores can become infected but serious complications like pneumonia or encephalitis (inflammation of the brain) are rare.

So, why would we immunise against chickenpox? Many Western countries say it is too expensive and have decided against it. Countries that opt to immunise do so mainly because people who are immunocompromised can get severe chickenpox and even die from it, and because immunisation against chickenpox reduces the later risk of shingles.

The chickenpox vaccine is a live attenuated virus vaccine. It was developed in Japan and was commercially available from 1984. It was used in Japan and Korea from 1988 and in the United States from 1995, and was introduced into the routine immunisation schedule in Australia in 2003.

Since 2013, Australia has given varicella vaccine in the form of a new quadrivalent four-in-one measles-mumps-rubella-varicella (MMRV) vaccine at 18 months, which reduces by one the number of injections a child gets. The United States recommends a second dose of varicella vaccine to boost immunity, but Australian authorities have ruled that the second dose is a costly luxury and decline to pay the price asked by vaccine companies.

Human papillomavirus

Human papillomavirus (HPV) vaccines are some of the newest and most exciting to be introduced. The excitement is because these vaccines protect women against cancer of the cervix, one of the commonest cancers for women after breast cancer.

Yet, as I will discuss in later chapters, HPV immunisation is controversial in many parts of the world. The cervix is the doorway to the womb, and anything to do with sex excites controversy.

Fortunately, Australians are more pragmatic than those in some other places. Australia was the first country in the world to introduce routine HPV immunisation of 12- to 13-year-old girls in a highly successful school-based program that started in 2007. It was also the first country to introduce routine HPV immunisation of 12- to 13-year-old boys in 2013, partly to protect against rare anal and penile cancers but mainly to protect girls, as with the rubella vaccine. The reward has been a significant fall in pre-malignant cervical lesions. In 2018, almost 1000 women in Australia will develop cervical cancer and just over 250 will die from it. Research predicts that due to HPV vaccine use, cervical cancer will become a 'rare cancer' in Australia in 2020 (defined as fewer than 6 new cases per 100,000 women annually) and fall below the elimination threshold of 4 per 100,000 by 2028, and that by 2066 Australia will be the first country in the world to eliminate cervical cancer.

Looking ahead

We often take immunisation for granted. But it is extraordinary to reflect on the diseases we can now prevent, and the way vaccines have transformed our lives in less than a century. Leading United States epidemiologists have estimated that 103 million cases of childhood disease have been prevented by immunisation since 1924 (95% of the infections that would have occurred without immunisation), and 26 million of them in the last decade alone (99% of the infections that would otherwise have occurred) – and that is just in the United States.

I call this the golden age of immunisation, although goodness knows what name others will come up with if we make even more progress. The present is exciting; the future could be breathtaking.

CHAPTER 8

Vaccines and cancer

Anti-immunisation groups sometimes assert that vaccines can cause cancer. But researchers have studied links between vaccines and cancers very carefully, and not only is there no suggestion that vaccines cause cancer, there is also the strongest possible evidence that two vaccines *prevent* cancer and at least one vaccine can *cure* cancer. The reason we can prevent cancer is that some cancers are caused by chronic virus infections, so preventing these infections can prevent cancer. The reason we can cure cancer is that we need our immune system to get rid of cancer, and some vaccines stimulate our immune system.

A critical question when thinking about cancers is why one person gets cancer and not another. The reasons are complex, but in simple terms they boil down to a combination of genetics, environment and time.

Legendary reggae musician Bob Marley died of malignant melanoma at just 36 years of age. Marley's father was a 50-year-old white itinerant overseer, Norval Marley, who falsely claimed to have been a captain in the British Caribbean army. He seduced Cedella, a 17-year-old Jamaican. Although he married her when she fell pregnant with Bob, he then ran away to Kingston and hardly ever visited his wife or son. Bob Marley later said bitterly that the only thing his father ever gave him was melanoma. He was correct.

White-skinned people have a rate of melanoma 20 times higher than black-skinned people, because melanin in the skin protects against melanoma: the darker the skin, the more melanin. Your skin colour is inherited from your parents, but the rate of melanoma is twice as high for white-skinned people in Australia as it is for white-skinned people in the United Kingdom, showing that increased exposure to sunlight increases the risk. Thus, your risk of getting melanoma depends on both your genes and your environment.

We know that the major environmental trigger for lung cancer is tobacco smoke. But in 18th century England, there were others. A London apothecary, John Hill, wrote that snuff could cause cancer of the lip, mouth and throat. Ten years later, a surgeon, Sir Percivall Pott, described chimney sweeps with scrotal cancer and made the link between the cancer and chimney soot, which stuck in their groin as they climbed chimneys near-naked. (He later identified Pott's disease of the spine, caused by tuberculosis, which can cause the hunchback gibbus deformity described in Chapter 5).

Tobacco smoke, snuff and soot are all examples of what we now call carcinogens, chemicals that cause chronic irritation and inflammation, and can change normal cells into abnormal ones. These changes can then progress to cancer.

To prevent cancer we also need a healthy immune system. Cancers are cells that reproduce abnormally and uncontrollably; immune cells can detect them, treat them as foreign and destroy them before they spread. Children born with severe immune deficiency, a genetic disorder, not only suffer from recurrent infections but also have a hugely increased risk of developing cancers. Just as their immune system does not recognise foreign organisms that cause infections, it also does not recognise cancer cells well.

Half the people living in an industrialised country will get cancer at some time in their life. The incidence of cancer has risen and continues to rise. The main reason for this is that we live longer: our immune system gradually deteriorates as we age, and over three-quarters of cancers occur in people over 60. One of the major reasons why we live longer is immunisation. There is an irony here: immunisations prolong our lives long enough for us to get cancer.

The antidote to the irony is that there are two cancers in humans that are potentially vaccine-preventable: liver cancer, which is usually caused by chronic hepatitis B virus infection; and cervical cancer, which is caused by human papillomaviruses. We also have vaccines that can be used to stimulate the immune system to treat cancer, such as BCG vaccine to treat bladder cancer, and there are more cancer-fighting vaccines on the way. This chapter will discuss some of these exciting developments.

Hepatitis B

James Nguyen was 41 years old when he came to the emergency department of the hospital where I was working. He was a charming, well-spoken, hardworking man with a wife and three children. He had been born in Vietnam and had immigrated to Australia with his parents when he was a teenager. Recently he had had some abdominal pain, vomited a few times and lost weight, which he put down to the vomiting and his poor appetite.

When I examined him, I found his liver was enlarged and tender and had a rather knobbly feel to it. Mr Nguyen had liver cancer. The reason he had liver cancer was that he was chronically infected with hepatitis B virus, almost certainly passed on to him at birth from his mother.

I was a 25-year-old doctor, not long qualified. I had to tell Mr Nguyen and his distraught wife and children about his diagnosis, and that it was too advanced for us to be able to operate on him.

Mr Nguyen died four weeks later, in his home, surrounded by his family. I have changed his name, but his story is true, and it still haunts me.

He did not need to die. More than half the cases of liver cancer – hepatocellular carcinoma or hepatoma – in the world are caused by chronic hepatitis B virus infection, and this infection is vaccine-preventable.

What is not generally appreciated is that if a pregnant woman has chronic hepatitis B infection, she can inadvertently pass the virus on to her baby around the time of birth. Babies who catch the infection at birth never get acute hepatitis. They usually remain asymptomatic into adulthood, if not for the whole of their life. But they never produce antibodies to the virus, which will stay in their liver till they die.

The scientific explanation of this is a phenomenon called immunological tolerance. The foetus of an infected pregnant woman is usually exposed to small amounts of hepatitis B in the womb, and the growing baby thinks the virus is part of itself, so becomes tolerant to it. The body should not make antibodies against itself; people who do so develop autoimmune diseases. Immunological tolerance was first described by the British scientists Sir Peter Medawar and Rupert Billingham, based on work by the Australian scientist Sir Macfarlane Burnet, and this discovery, so important for transplant surgery, won the three of them the Nobel Prize in 1960.

Although babies chronically infected with hepatitis B are asymptomatic, the virus lurking in their liver can start to cause chronic inflammation. This can lead to scarring called cirrhosis, which we usually associate with liver damage from chronic alcohol abuse, but which can occur in people with chronic viral infection who drink no alcohol. As Mr Nguyen's story demonstrates, the virus can also cause cancer of the liver.

Before the availability of vaccines, a quarter to a third of people with chronic hepatitis B infection died young from cirrhosis or liver cancer. In countries like Indonesia, Thailand, Cambodia, South Korea, Macau, Taiwan, China and Vietnam, in the 1970s and 1980s before routine hepatitis B immunisation was introduced, an astonishing one in seven children (15%) were infected at birth. Even today, there are 350 million people in the world with chronic infection, and about 600,000 of them die from hepatitis B complications every year.

Thanks to the vaccine, though, people like Mr Nguyen need never be infected at birth and need never have to suffer the way he did. The virus responsible for hepatitis B was discovered in 1965 – not by the many virologists and cancer specialists trying vainly to find a virus that caused cancer, but by a Philadelphia biochemist called Baruch Blumberg. This discovery would win him the Nobel Prize, although, initially at least, his discovery owed a great deal to serendipity.

Blumberg was interested in how genetic variations might make populations more susceptible to diseases, and this was his excuse to travel the world, from Africa to Asia to Australia, collecting blood samples from remote tribespeople and testing their blood for proteins called antigens. Blumberg found a blood antigen present in some Australian Aborigines that was also found in some people in Africa and Asia, but rarely in people in America or Europe. Blumberg thought this was a genetic factor, and called it 'Australia antigen'. His studies showed a link with liver cirrhosis, and he thought he had found an inherited protein antigen that predisposed people to chronic liver inflammation. However, one day in 1966, an American patient whom Blumberg had been studying who was known to have no Australia antigen suddenly developed acute hepatitis, and at the same time tested positive for Australia antigen. Clearly, the protein antigen was not inherited but one that the man had just acquired.

Blumberg's real achievement was to labour diligently to identify this protein. Within a few years, his laboratory had shown that the protein antigen was produced by a virus, which he purified and called the hepatitis B virus. The Australia antigen was renamed hepatitis B surface antigen (HBs), because it sat on the surface of cells. By 1979, Blumberg's team had developed the first ever hepatitis B vaccine from purified surface antigen.

A critical finding was that patients in Africa and Southeast Asia with liver cancer were far more likely to have chronic hepatitis B virus infection than patients *without* liver cancer. One possible explanation was that chronic hepatitis B caused chronic scarring (cirrhosis) that could lead to liver cancer. The implication was that a vaccine that prevented hepatitis B infection could prevent many liver cancers.

Today the newborn babies of women who are chronically infected with hepatitis B respond well to the vaccine. The difference between this response and the baby's response to natural infection is that the vaccine contains aluminium (alum) as an adjuvant to boost the baby's immune response and thus overcome the tolerance. This illustrates the importance of vaccine adjuvants; people who worry unduly about trace amounts of aluminium in vaccines do not usually understand that the vaccines would not work without them.

In 1984, Taiwan became the first country in the world to introduce routine neonatal (newborn) hepatitis B immunisation. Within 13 years, the incidence of liver cancer in children aged six to nine dropped from 0.52 to 0.13 per 100,000, a fall of 75%. This is strong evidence. Most European countries (47 of 53) and some countries in Southeast Asia have introduced universal hepatitis B vaccines.

The WHO has set a goal for hepatitis B vaccination to become part of universal childhood vaccination programs in all countries. By the end of 2016, 186 countries had introduced nationwide vaccination, and by 2015, the WHO estimated that 84% of the world's children had been immunised, 114 of the world's countries had achieved better than 90% coverage, and only six countries were below 50% coverage.

Hepatitis B is a virus that causes misery, cancer and early death, and which we will eventually eliminate from the world by immunisation.

Human papillomaviruses

In 1913, George Papanicolaou arrived in New York by boat, to seek his fortune. He had trained in medicine in Athens and

Munich, yet now he was penniless with no job, so he resorted to selling carpets on 33rd Street. Later he applied to Cornell University and was employed in the research laboratory, investigating the menstrual cycle of guinea-pigs. He learned from scratch how to obtain cells from the female guinea-pig's cervix – an eye-watering process (I shall spare you the details).

Papanicolaou was fascinated by how he could tell the stage of the menstrual cycle from the cells obtained by these cervical smears. He started to experiment on humans. I can't resist adding that his wife was his first guinea-pig: Maria submitted to daily cervical smears while George perfected his technique. When you talk about long-suffering wives, do bear Maria in mind.

Cervical smears were an invasive way of predicting the menstrual cycle. But Papanicolaou started to examine smears from women with different gynaecological conditions and found that women with cervical cancer shed bizarre cells that he could see when he did a smear.

In 1928 he published a paper named 'New Cancer Diagnosis', giving the first description of what we now call the Pap smear. Yet it took over 20 years of research for Papanicolaou to crystallise his thoughts. It was only in 1950, when challenged at a Christmas party as to the use of his smears, that Papanicolaou was able to give voice to his dreams: the real purpose of Pap smears was to detect early pre-malignant changes and intervene before the cells became cancerous.

Two years later, 150,000 women in Shelby County, Tennessee, were given a Pap smear. Of these 555 had cervical cancer, while another 557 had early, precancerous lesions. (These could be removed by a simple surgical procedure called a cone biopsy, because it involved removing a cone-shaped chunk of tissue.)

These women were well and symptom-free and were on average 20 years younger than those with cancer. The Pap smear had the potential to detect cervical cancers 20 or more years earlier than previous screening methods.

Regular Pap smears have undoubtedly prevented many thousands of cases of cervical cancer, but they cannot prevent all. On current figures, more than 900 women in Australia will develop cervical cancer in 2018, and 250 women will die from it. In the United States there will be in excess of 13,000 cases and more than 4000 deaths.

Harald zur Hausen is a German virologist who moved to the United States in 1965 to collaborate with Werner and Gertrude Henle in the virus laboratory of the Children's Hospital of Philadelphia. The Henles were married German Jews who had fled Nazi Germany in 1936. Their field of interest was oncoviruses, viruses that could cause cancer. In 1968 Werner Henle became the first person to show that a virus could change normal cells into cancer cells, by using Epstein-Barr virus to infect normal white blood cells.

In 1976, zur Hausen published a paper hypothesising that human papillomaviruses were an important cause of cervical cancer. Papillomaviruses are wart viruses: some cause skin warts or plantar warts (verrucas); some are sexually transmitted and can cause ano-genital warts; and some can cause mouth papillomas. In 1983 and 1984, zur Hausen and his team identified two human papillomaviruses, HPV-16 and HPV-18, in specimens of cervical cancer. The following year he cloned HPV-16 and HPV-18. Although this did not prove that human papillomaviruses cause cervical cancer, subsequent studies showed that he was right. Harald zur Hausen was awarded a Nobel Prize in 2008.

Harald zur Hausen's discovery paved the way for the development of vaccines to prevent human papillomavirus infection. The first vaccine against HPV was developed by Ian Frazer and Jian Zhou at the University of Queensland.

Ian Frazer was born in Glasgow, as was my scientist father, Alick. Like my father before him, Frazer travelled to the Walter & Eliza Hall Institute in Melbourne to enhance his training. On sabbatical to Cambridge University in 1989, Frazer met Jian Zhou, a younger virologist who had trained in China. Frazer persuaded Jian to join him in Queensland. They used DNA-recombining techniques to produce virus-like particles that do not contain any viral genetic material, so are non-infectious. Jian died in 1999 before seeing their work come to full fruition. (Sadly, he died from complications of chronic hepatitis B infection, which, as we've just heard, can cause cancer and can be prevented by immunisation.)

Two pharmaceutical companies led the way in bringing HPV vaccines to market: Merck in the United States introduced Gardasil, and GlaxoSmithKline (GSK) in the United Kingdom produced Cervarix. Cervarix provided immunisation against two strains of HPV, while Gardasil protected against four strains.

In 2007, Professor Suzanne Garland of the Royal Women's Hospital in Melbourne published the results of a three-year trial of over 5000 women aged 16 to 24. Half the women had received three doses of Gardasil and half had received three doses of a placebo. Pre-malignant cervical cell changes developed in 65 women who had received the placebo but in none of the women given the vaccine. However, the vaccine did not protect women already infected with HPV. These results, while impressive, clearly show that HPV vaccines should be given *before* women are infected. Merck has now developed a newer version of Gardasil vaccine that protects against five additional HPV strains.

The evidence strongly suggests that HPV infection is the major cause of cervical cancer, and that HPV vaccine has the potential to prevent a huge proportion of all cervical cancers. Scientists can also detect HPV in anal cancer, penile cancer and oropharyngeal cancer (cancer of the throat), but they are less certain that HPV actually causes those cancers, and therefore less certain that HPV vaccine can prevent them.

Globally, it is estimated that over 500,000 new cases of cancer a year are caused by chronic HPV infections and can potentially be prevented by vaccines. Eventually we will probably have HPV vaccines that will almost eradicate cervical cancer. How remarkable is that?

Some fascinating ethical issues have arisen with HPV vaccines, however. One issue (which will be dealt with in Chapter 13) is the use of HPV vaccines on boys. Another issue (which we'll hear about in Chapter 12) surrounds the way the United States company Merck's vaccine, Gardasil, was marketed in the United States.

A third issue is the question of cost. The initial price of the HPV vaccine was high, around US$450 for a course of three doses. Merck and GSK said they needed to recoup the huge costs of vaccine development. When Gardasil and Cervarix were considered by the Pharmaceutical Benefits Advisory Committee in Australia, it found the high price was justified by the considerable benefits. The price paid in Australia is completely prohibitive for developing countries, but once uptake was guaranteed in some resource-rich countries, both companies supplied their vaccines at a fraction of the price to resource-poor countries.

It seems eminently reasonable that rich countries should pay a high but affordable price that in turn allows the companies to minimise costs in poor countries. Pharmaceutical companies can never be accused of excessive altruism, but this pragmatic equity deserves praise. The lowest current prices are around US$12.80 a dose in Brazil and South Africa. Many countries still cannot afford that price, and Gavi, the Vaccine Alliance – funded by the Bill and Melinda Gates Foundation – subsidises some of the poorest countries.

By 2014, 33.6% of all women aged 20 to 40 in wealthy countries had received a full course of HPV vaccine, compared with only 1 in 40 (2.7%) in low- or middle-income countries. An estimated 47 million people worldwide had been fully vaccinated against HPV by 2015, thus preventing 379,000 cases of cervical cancer and 156,000 deaths. Australia leads the way: it was the first country in the world to introduce a routine school-based program for girls, in 2007, and the first to immunise all boys, beginning in 2013; vaccinations were also offered to some older women. Projections suggest that Australia will be the first country in the world to eliminate cervical cancer, and possibly within your lifetime if not mine. What a thrilling prospect: to prevent thousands of young women dying from cancer through immunisation.

Helicobacter pylori

Barry Marshall was born in the goldfields town of Kalgoorlie in Western Australia. He trained as a doctor in Perth. In the early 1980s he became interested in gastritis (inflammation of the stomach) and peptic ulcers. At the time, the medical community was convinced that stress and lifestyle factors such as smoking were the cause of stomach ulcers.

Barry's Perth pathologist colleague Robin Warren observed curved, rod-like bacteria in the stomach lining of patients with gastritis. Barry succeeded in growing them, but was unable to infect laboratory animals with them. Barry and Robin called the bacteria *Helicobacter pylori*, meaning spiral stomach bacteria, and published their findings in a letter to the prestigious journal *The Lancet*.

Some letter. Their international colleagues thought the bacteria Barry and Robin were seeing down the microscope were not real, but were artefacts induced when processing the specimens. Even if the organisms were real, most critics doubted they could survive in stomach acid.

Desperate to convince the sceptics, Barry Marshall let someone put a tube down his throat to perform a biopsy on his stomach, which proved he had not previously been infected with *Helicobacter pylori*, then drank a suspension of the organism. Over the next two weeks he developed abdominal pains, and submitted himself to two more biopsies to prove he had gastritis, and to grow the organism from his stomach. He then took antibiotics, which cleared the infection and his symptoms. The mind boggles at the things some people (but not many) will do for science.

We now know *Helicobacter pylori* causes over 90% of duodenal ulcers and up to 80% of gastric ulcers, and is also associated with gastric cancer. It can usually be eradicated with antibiotics. In 2005, Barry Marshall and Robin Warren were awarded a Nobel Prize for their discovery, which has revolutionised the management and prevention of stomach and duodenal ulcers.

Despite intense research, no effective vaccine is yet available commercially against *Helicobacter pylori*. But when one is finally developed it will prevent many thousands of cases of stomach cancer.

Other vaccines that treat cancer

As we've learned, BCG vaccine is a live attenuated vaccine developed to prevent tuberculosis and made from the cow TB organism *Mycobacterium bovis*.

Since the 1970s, the non-specific immune stimulation that BCG vaccine provides has often been used to treat patients with bladder cancer. The initial treatment for adults is usually to use a scope to enter the bladder and burn away the cancer. Bladder cancers can also be resected (cut out). However, the cancer has a strong likelihood of recurring, often repeatedly so, despite multiple attempts to burn or cut it away.

We need a working immune system if we are to recover from cancer, just as we need it to recover from infections. BCG vaccine, instilled directly through a catheter into the bladder, works in a non-specific way (nothing to do with its protection against TB) to stimulate immune cells in the bladder, and the increased immunity allows the cells to eliminate the cancer. BCG vaccine reduces the risk of recurrence of bladder cancer by about 20%. If at first that does not sound all that impressive, for many thousands of sufferers it means the difference between having repeated operations for recurrences of bladder cancer and being cured.

Sipuleucel-T was the first cancer vaccine to be licensed. It was approved by the United States Food and Drug Administration

(FDA) in 2010 to treat some men with metastatic prostate cancer (prostate cancer that has already spread). It stimulates the immune response to an antigen (foreign substance) called prostatic acid phosphatase. Men with one type of metastatic prostate cancer given Sipuleucel-T in a clinical trial lived just over four months longer than men not given the drug. Many people see an extra four months as being very worthwhile to get their affairs in order and say their farewells.

On target

We can now prevent children and adults from getting liver cancer using hepatitis B vaccine, and we can prevent women from getting cancer of the cervix using HPV vaccines. We can also reduce recurrence of bladder cancer using BCG vaccine, and extend the lives of men with prostate cancer.

In the future, scientists hope to develop many more cancer vaccines, including vaccines that target cancers caused by virus infections, as well as vaccines that stimulate the immune system to fight off cancer.

CHAPTER 9

Vaccines and pregnancy

Riley was the second child of Catherine and Greg Hughes. Riley was a normal, healthy baby, born in February 2015 in Perth. When he was three weeks old, he developed a runny nose and occasional cough. The family doctor said it was only a virus, but Riley became sleepy and went off his feeds.

His parents took him to hospital, where he was found to have pneumonia due to whooping cough. His breathing deteriorated despite intensive care, and after five days in hospital, Riley Hughes died.

Riley was 32 days old. His parents did not know that a local whooping cough outbreak had just started, nor that immunising pregnant women in the last three months of pregnancy reduces the risk that their newborn babies will catch whooping cough.

Riley's parents posted a video online that was taken in his last days of life, showing him coughing uncontrollably and going blue in the face. They started a movement, Light for Riley, to inform others about the benefits of immunising pregnant women against whooping cough in the third trimester of pregnancy, to try to prevent anyone else from having to go through the same tragedy as them.

Pregnant women are at increased risk from infections because their immune system does not work as well as normal. This reduced immunity is necessary to prevent the immune system from rejecting the foetus as 'foreign', which could lead to miscarriage. Thus, a pregnant woman infected with a virus such as chickenpox or influenza may develop a life-threatening disease.

One reason for immunising a woman before or even during pregnancy is to protect her. A second reason is so that she will produce antibodies that can cross the placenta and protect her infant against congenital infection (being born already infected).

Some infections, such as rubella, can pass through the placenta and infect the foetus during pregnancy, causing severe congenital defects. Congenital rubella can be prevented by pre-pregnancy rubella vaccine. Babies are also at risk of catching potentially severe infections at the time of birth, such as tetanus, or soon after birth, such as whooping cough, as Riley did.

Doctors may be reluctant to recommend pregnancy vaccines for fear that the vaccines will harm the unborn child. This is a perfectly rational fear. We know that things that happen to women during pregnancy can affect their foetus. Almost everyone knows about the malformations of babies' arms and legs caused when pregnant women took thalidomide to prevent morning sickness during the 1950s. Fortunately, there is good evidence that the vaccines currently recommended during pregnancy are safe as well as effective.

This chapter will discuss maternal immunisation *before* pregnancy to prevent congenital rubella syndrome and neonatal tetanus, and *during* pregnancy to protect both the mother and her newborn infant against influenza and whooping cough.

Rubella

Rubella vaccine is a live attenuated viral vaccine. As we have seen, it is given to both girls and boys to prevent rubella circulating and thus stop non-immune pregnant women catching rubella. In this way it prevents congenital rubella syndrome. It is not recommended in pregnancy because of the theoretical risk that it might cause congenital rubella syndrome. However, of the more than 3500 women globally who have been inadvertently given rubella vaccine just before they became pregnant or in early pregnancy and elected to continue with their pregnancy, not a single one has had a baby with congenital rubella syndrome.

The breakthrough in understanding rubella and congenital rubella syndrome came during World War II. Norman McAlister Gregg was an Australian ophthalmologist who played cricket and tennis for New South Wales and was later knighted. He worked at the same hospital as I do, the Children's Hospital at Westmead, then known as the Royal Alexandra Hospital for Children, in Sydney, making him a local hero as well as an international one. Gregg had an inquiring mind and was interested in everything, particularly his patients. He was also a kind man, who kept a tin of biscuits in his office for the children who visited him.

In 1941, Gregg suddenly started seeing a large number of newborn infants with eye defects, particularly cataracts. While pondering the cause, Gregg overheard two mothers in the waiting room saying they had both had German measles early in their pregnancy. There had been a rubella epidemic in Sydney during the spring and summer before the babies were born.

Intrigued, and wondering if the cataracts could be due to maternal rubella, Gregg inquired among other mothers of affected infants in his practice, as well as those of his colleagues. Gregg himself had seen 13 affected babies; his colleagues told him about another 65. The majority of the mothers – 68 of the 78 whose babies were affected – remembered having a rubella-like illness with a rash in early pregnancy.

On 15 October 1941, Gregg delivered a paper called 'Congenital Cataract Following German Measles in the Mother' to the Ophthalmological Society of Australia. The paper was later published in the society's journal. The Sydney press reported Gregg's findings on the Monday morning after the meeting, and before lunchtime the same day two mothers telephoned Gregg to say they had had rubella in early pregnancy and their children were deaf but were otherwise well.

We now know that if a woman catches rubella early in the first trimester (first three months), her baby may have the full congenital rubella syndrome, whereas if she is infected between 14 and 17 weeks, the infant may be deaf but without other defects. This is because the rubella virus attacks organs at a critical stage of their development in the foetus: the eyes, brain and heart develop early in the first trimester and the ears a bit later.

Gregg's discoveries were doubted until the same clinical findings were documented in an outbreak in the United States. As the first person to recognise that the organisms infecting a pregnant woman could cross the placenta and harm the foetus, Gregg had achieved something truly remarkable. He is a wonderful example of a physician – an eye surgeon, at that – who listened to mothers, thought about what they said and followed through with intelligent inquiry. Gregg's observation, the first recognition of congenital rubella syndrome, helped hasten the development of rubella vaccine, which has in turn prevented the deaths of many thousands of infants.

Rubella virus was isolated in the early 1960s, and by the end of that decade vaccines were available. Gregg was honoured in his lifetime, but was always a modest and unassuming man. When he received an invitation from an Italian pathologist, Professor Alfonso Giordano, to be nominated for a Nobel Prize, Sir Norman Gregg replied:

> I must confess that it comes as a great surprise and rather
> a shock that my name should even be considered ... I feel it
> only fair to you to inform you that I have really no serious
> publications except those on rubella as I have found very
> little time or inclination for writing during a very busy life.

Other doctors soon recognised that congenital rubella syndrome was a devastating condition, and could cause microcephaly (a small head), severe intellectual impairment, blindness, deafness and congenital heart disease. Babies with severe congenital rubella syndrome who cannot see and cannot hear become 'locked in'; it is almost impossible to communicate with them. These are some of the most heartbreakingly damaged children a paediatrician ever sees.

Before immunisation, rubella epidemics occurred every six to nine years, and major pandemics about every 10 to 30 years. Epidemiologists estimate that 10% of all pregnant women developed rubella infection in the last major world pandemic from 1963 to 1965, and 30% of their infants developed congenital rubella syndrome. In the United States, over 12 million people caught rubella during that pandemic, as a result of which 11,000 pregnant women miscarried, over 2000 babies died soon after birth, and 20,000 infants were born with major congenital defects. In recent years, though, there has been on average fewer than one case each year of congenital rubella syndrome in the whole of the United States.

Congenital rubella syndrome has all but been eliminated from first-world countries thanks to rubella vaccine. National rubella vaccine programs had been established in 147 countries by the end of 2015.

But there is no room for complacency. Less than half the world can afford routine rubella vaccine, global coverage is only around 46%, and the WHO estimates that worldwide 100,000 babies a year are still born with congenital rubella syndrome.

Tetanus

We learned in Chapter 7 how tetanus is passed from the soil, and about its prevalence in newborns in Africa. Newborns can be infected by tetanus at or soon after birth if their umbilicus is not adequately cleaned, and particularly if animal dung or even ghee (clarified butter) is applied to their umbilicus, as is the cultural practice in some countries. The bacterium *Clostridium tetani* that causes tetanus often lives in the intestines of cattle and horses and is found in their dung.

A newborn baby who develops tetanus is almost certain to die. Yet babies can be almost completely protected if their mothers are fully immunised against tetanus, because the mother makes protective antibodies that cross the placenta and enter the baby's bloodstream. Maternal immunisation prevents 94% of cases of neonatal tetanus.

For 150 years on the island of St Kilda in Scotland's Outer Hebrides, more than two-thirds of all babies born died from tetanus within two weeks of birth. After a few days they would stop being able to suck; they were said to have a sardonic smile, which was no smile at all, but spasm of the face muscles. The disease was called 'the sickness of eight days'. Between 1855 and 1876, 41 of the 56 babies born on St Kilda died. In 1885, a *Glasgow Herald* journalist, Robert Connell, wrote: 'A great gun of the Free Church was not ashamed to say that this lock-jaw was a wise device of the Almighty for keeping the population within the resources of the island.'

In 1890, a St Kilda minister, the Reverend Angus Fiddes, discovered that the local midwife, who was called the 'knee-woman', used to 'clean' each newborn baby's umbilicus with ruby-red oil obtained from a local seabird, the fulmar. The oil was kept in a gourd made from the dried stomach of a bird known locally as a solan goose, although we would call it a gannet. The gourd was never cleaned.

On learning all this, Fiddes threw the gourd over the cliff and ended the disastrous spectre of neonatal tetanus that had haunted women on the island. He persuaded public health nurses from Glasgow to educate the lay midwife about modern birthing practices. No cases of neonatal tetanus occurred on St Kilda after 1891.

Neonatal tetanus occurs when spores contaminate the cut umbilical stump. On St Kilda, the midwife's gourd was presumably contaminated with tetanus spores. In some African countries, neonatal tetanus is known as 'no-suck disease' and is acquired through a traditional practice of putting mud on the umbilical stump. (As I mentioned in Chapter 7, I have witnessed this myself.) Mud of course contains dung, which harbours lots of spores of *Clostridium tetani*. In India, it was more common to use ghee (clarified butter), but this too could be contaminated with tetanus spores and cause neonatal tetanus.

The WHO estimates that 787,000 newborns died of neonatal tetanus in 1988. This stimulated a campaign to reduce and eventually eliminate neonatal tetanus, through increased immunisation of girls and pregnant women, and through improved umbilical cord hygiene.

While there were initially some problems in implementing the recommended strategies, the WHO has now made considerable progress. In 2015, the WHO estimates that 34,000 newborns died from neonatal tetanus, a 96% reduction from the late 1980s. By the end of 2016, only 18 countries had not succeeded in eliminating neonatal tetanus.

Influenza

Influenza is a respiratory virus that spreads in the air through coughs and sneezes. Hippocrates described influenza's hacking cough, runny nose, sore throat, fever, headache, aches and pains about 2500 years ago. The name comes from the Latin *influentia*, 'influence', because medieval physicians thought the huge outbreaks that came around without fail year after year were influenced by the movements of the heavenly spheres.

Influenza virus still kills up to half a million humans every year. As we saw in Chapter 1, a worldwide influenza pandemic can wipe out millions of people in a few weeks.

Infection can cause a viral pneumonia, which can sometimes be complicated by bacteria, causing a 'super-infection' (one infection on top of the other). Influenza infection also causes the body to release proteins such as interferon, which help fight off the influenza virus but themselves cause high fever, shivers and shakes (rigors), headache and severe muscle aches and pains debilitating enough to render healthy youngsters bed-bound for a week or two.

Pneumonia is the usual cause of death if flu proves fatal, but an influenza infection can also affect the heart. Young adults occasionally die from myocarditis if they exercise when they have influenza. People who have a heart attack (myocardial infarction) are twice as likely to have had a recent influenza-like illness as people who do not suffer a heart attack. Even children are not totally safe from death: a small number of previously normal healthy children around two to four years old die suddenly from influenza each year.

Pregnant women are more than twice as likely to be hospitalised if they catch influenza as non-pregnant women of the same age. The infants of pregnant women who catch influenza are significantly more likely to be born premature or underweight.

A large randomised controlled trial in Bangladesh showed that inactivated killed influenza vaccine protected pregnant women and also protected more than half their infants from catching influenza in their first six months after birth. A similar trial in South Africa found that the vaccine protected about half of all pregnant women against influenza, and their infants were half as likely to catch the virus.

There are a couple of myths about influenza vaccines. The first myth, propagated by some doctors, is that the vaccine does not work. It is true that the vaccine does not prevent *all* influenza. The proteins in the virus change a little each year, a phenomenon known as antigenic drift. For this reason, a new influenza vaccine is produced each year under the aegis of the WHO, based on the likely circulating strains of influenza. The vaccine will contain three or four different strains. In practice the match between the vaccine and the strains that actually circulate varies from year to year, so the vaccine's efficacy varies too. Critics often point out correctly that influenza vaccine is less effective than vaccines against diseases like measles, but sometimes we have to live with imperfection, until we can do better.

It is also true that people with weakened immune systems, such as cancer patients and the elderly, do not respond as well to the vaccine, even though they are the people who need it most because influenza is more severe if your immune system is weakened. (Stronger influenza vaccines are available now and may be the answer – we'll look at influenza and the elderly in Chapter 10.)

The second myth is that influenza vaccines actually *cause* influenza. In fact, most of them are inactivated influenza vaccines, which contain only proteins and so are incapable of causing influenza.

There are a number of possible reasons for feeling like these vaccines have given you the flu. It could be chance: you may be unlucky enough to catch a respiratory virus infection soon after receiving the flu vaccine. It could also be that your body's immune response to the vaccine causes fever and aches, although controlled studies show this is not much more common than if you are given a placebo.

The influenza vaccine is extremely safe during pregnancy. Inactivated influenza vaccine has been recommended for pregnant women in the United States since 1960, so there is a long history of its use and good data to show that it does not cause problems to mother, foetus or newborn baby. Influenza vaccine has been given safely to Australian women for over 20 years, and the vaccine is in the lowest risk category for medicines in pregnancy.

Several studies have shown that the vaccine does not increase the rate of miscarriage, stillbirth or birth defects. In fact, a meta-analysis (combining the results of all similar studies) found that pregnant women given influenza vaccine were less likely to have a stillbirth than those *not* given the vaccine. Influenza vaccine is also extremely cheap, at around $10 a dose or less.

For pregnant women, being protected by influenza vaccine is far better than remaining unvaccinated.

Whooping cough

As already discussed, whooping cough (pertussis) is a life-threatening disease in the first months of life. Between 1980 and 1989, the United States reported 77 deaths from pertussis, of which 61 were infants under three months old.

I discussed the difference between whole-cell and acellular pertussis vaccines in Chapter 7. The acellular pertussis vaccines currently used in much of the industrialised world are less likely than the whole-cell vaccines to cause adverse effects such as fever. On the downside, the protection they provide is relatively short-lived. This is why pertussis continues to circulate.

At least two, preferably three, doses of pertussis vaccine are needed for adequate protection. But clinical trials show that newborn babies do not respond to the vaccine. The earliest time when babies can be immunised is at six weeks, and the second dose is given between 10 weeks and three or four months of age.

It is not surprising that most infants catch whooping cough from a parent, sibling or grandparent. One way of trying to protect infants has been to immunise their close relatives, a strategy given the touching name 'cocooning'. This practice was adopted briefly in some places, including Australia and the United States, but unfortunately it has been difficult to prove that it works well.

A more effective intervention is to immunise mothers in late pregnancy. Pertussis vaccine is rarely marketed on its own nowadays, but is usually combined with diphtheria and tetanus vaccines into the triple DTP vaccine, or sometimes with other vaccines.

An average of four people die of whooping cough each year in the United Kingdom, but 14 babies under three months old died in an outbreak in 2012. In October 2012, the United Kingdom Department of Health introduced an emergency program to administer a vaccine containing tetanus, diphtheria, pertussis and polio vaccines (Tdap-IPV) to all pregnant women between 28 and 32 weeks' gestation.

A study of over 26,000 pregnant women, of whom almost two-thirds received the vaccine, showed that it was over 90% effective in preventing pertussis in infants aged less than two months old whose mothers were immunised at least a week prior to delivery. The United Kingdom has continued the program and it has been 95% effective in reducing infant deaths from pertussis.

A safe option

Immunising mothers-to-be during pregnancy has been shown to be very effective in protecting their newborn babies against some potentially devastating infections. The vaccines also protect the women themselves. Despite understandable concerns about the safety of vaccines in pregnancy, large studies have shown that the vaccines currently recommended in pregnancy are extremely safe as well as effective.

CHAPTER 10

Vaccines for the elderly

Increasing life expectancy has revealed the extent to which our immunity wanes with age: a phenomenon sometimes given the disrespectful name of 'immunosenescence'. Our immunity gets worse with time in the same way as we lose our memory; it forgets as much as our brain does.

Doctors can boost waning immunity in the elderly with vaccines, but we are faced with the obstacle that our immune system responds less well to vaccines as we grow older.

Shingles (zoster)

As we learned in Chapter 7, shingles (zoster) is a blistering, painful skin eruption, usually on one side of the body, caused by the reactivation of the chickenpox virus. The incidence of shingles increases with age: about a quarter of all people will have at least one attack of shingles in their lifetime, rising to half of all people who reach 85 years old.

Shingles and chickenpox are both caused by the varicella zoster virus (VZV). When we recover from chickenpox, the virus does not go away but lies dormant (latent) in our nerve cells. The rash may even recur in the same place in some people. Things known to increase the risk of shingles are stress and other impairments of the immune system, such as cancer, some drugs or old age.

Grandparents in close contact with young children are less likely to develop shingles than people of the same age who have no contact with young children. When children catch chickenpox for the first time, they expose others to it, including grandparents. This acts like a vaccine, boosting the elderly person's immune response to the virus and making it less likely that they will develop shingles. This is because a healthy immune system 'remembers' the chickenpox virus and keeps it in check.

The severity of shingles also increases with age. For reasons nobody has ever been able to explain, children almost never get post-herpetic neuralgia – the severe, prolonged nerve pain following a bout of shingles – whereas the condition can devastate the physical, psychological, functional and social lives of the elderly. This in turn may precipitate major depression; some patients even commit suicide.

As our population has aged, the need to boost immunity with a zoster vaccine has become increasingly apparent. The first zoster vaccines were really just highly concentrated varicella vaccine; they contained the same live attenuated VZV virus, grown in the same way, but 14 times as much of it. A new zoster vaccine made from purified VZV protein plus an adjuvant has been used in recent clinical trials. Studies of both types of vaccine show that people over 60 years old given zoster vaccine were half as likely as those given a placebo to develop zoster over the following three years.

There are problems with zoster vaccines, however. One is cost: the current vaccine is very expensive, although in the light of the often life-wrecking human cost of zoster, several countries, including the United States, the United Kingdom and Australia, have assessed it as cost-effective and elected to pay for it. Another problem is that because of waning immunity (immunosenescence, if you must), the vaccine becomes less effective with age, yet the highest incidence of zoster occurs among older people. Deciding on the optimum age to give the vaccine – based on both waning efficacy and increasing incidence – involves complex calculations. We know protection from the vaccine is likely to wane with time and the VZV virus stays in our nerves forever, so we may find we will need to give extra booster doses of zoster vaccine as people age, incurring additional expense.

In 2013, England introduced routine herpes zoster vaccine for adults aged 70, with a phased catch-up program for those aged 71 to 79. After three years, there were an estimated 17,000 fewer episodes of herpes zoster and 3300 fewer episodes of post-herpetic neuralgia in a population of 5.5 million.

When varicella immunisation is introduced for the whole child population, as has been done in the United States, Canada, Australia and several countries in Europe and the Middle East, chickenpox does not circulate nearly as much as previously. There is a risk that decreased exposure to natural chickenpox will mean the elderly will have less boosting of their immunity and be more likely to develop shingles. Because of this concern, the United Kingdom has not introduced routine childhood varicella immunisation.

The British fears are supported by data from Australia showing a slow but steady rise in the incidence of shingles since 2005, when routine childhood varicella immunisation was introduced. On a more optimistic note, modelling predicts that the incidence of shingles will plateau in Australia after 30 years, then decline to levels far lower than without varicella immunisation. In the United States, though, shingles incidence appears unaffected by the introduction of chickenpox vaccine. Modelling is not a perfect science and what happens in the real world can vary depending on unexpected or unexplained circumstances.

Influenza

People of any age from infancy to old age can die from seasonal influenza, but mortality is highest in the elderly.

There is strong evidence that older people can derive some protection from annual influenza immunisation. Most first-world countries recognise this by paying for annual influenza immunisation for the elderly.

Scientists have made various attempts to improve the vaccine's effectiveness. One is the manufacture of a live attenuated influenza vaccine that is given intranasally (squirted up the nose). This vaccine works well in children but has no advantages over the killed vaccine in the elderly, and is not used for them. (For safety reasons, it is not used for pregnant women either.)

Other approaches have been to add adjuvants that boost the immune response (adjuvanted influenza vaccines) and to increase the dose of antigens (high-dose inactivated influenza vaccines). Both these vaccines improve protection by about a quarter, but have a higher cost. As we heard in Chapter 1, the elderly can also be protected against influenza by immunising schoolchildren, through herd immunity.

In 2018, the Australian Government paid for all people over 65 years old to receive either an adjuvanted or a high-dose influenza vaccine for free. The long-term routine use of these vaccines will depend on balancing the increased protection against the increased cost. Since influenza vaccines are unlike most vaccines, in that they have to be given annually, any variation in cost is a recurring one.

Pneumococcus

Sir William Osler (1849–1919) was a famous Canadian physician who is sometimes known as the Father of Modern Medicine. He once called pneumonia 'the friend of the aged' – often expressed as 'the old man's friend' – because of the disease's propensity to hasten demise.

This begs the question of whether you *want* your 'friend' to help you die; you might prefer to hang around a little longer. (It also begs the question of why the old man's friend excludes women.) Osler worked before antibiotics or vaccines against pneumonia were available; nowadays, the fatalistic concept of pneumonia as a good exit strategy for the elderly is rarely felt to be appropriate.

As we heard in Chapter 7, the influenza virus is a major cause of pneumonia in the elderly. But another important cause is a bacterium called *Streptococcus pneumoniae*, or pneumococcus (from the Greek *pneumon*, lung, and *kokkos*, grain or seed). There are many different strains of pneumococcus, depending on their different outer sugar capsule. Pneumococci tend to be seen in pairs, so used to be called diplococci ('double seeds').

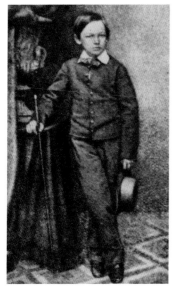

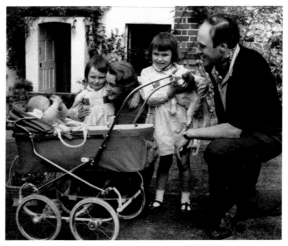

Author Roald Dahl with his wife, Patricia Neal, and their three children – from left to right, Theo, Tessa and Olivia. Seven-year-old Olivia died of measles in 1962. *(Alamy)*

Willie Lincoln, son of Abraham Lincoln, who died of typhoid, aged 11, in 1862. *(Library of Congress)*

A miniature from the Toggenburg Bible (Switzerland), dating from 1411, showing smallpox victims and a priest trying to treat them, probably with herbs – aromatherapy was then a common remedy. *(Wikimedia Commons)*

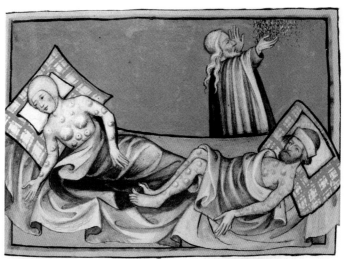

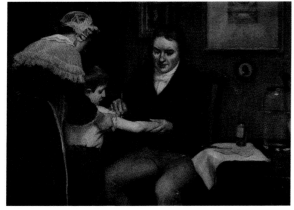

Edward Jenner performing his first smallpox vaccination, on eight-year-old James Phipps, on 14 May 1796; painting by Ernest Board (1877–1934). *(Wellcome Collection: CC BY)*

In his famous 1802 cartoon *The Cow-Pock – or – the Wonderful Effects of the New Inoculation!*, English satirist James Gillray depicted cows emerging from the bodies of people being vaccinated with the new cowpox vaccine. *(Wellcome Collection: CC BY)*

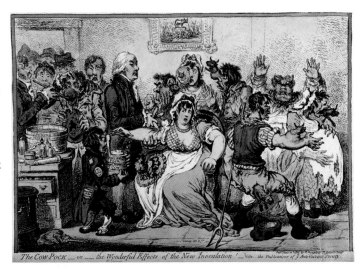

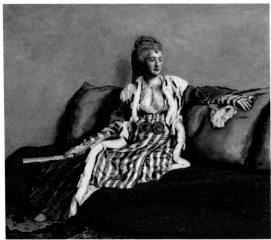

Lady Montagu in Turkish Dress by Jean-Etienne Liotard, c. 1756; Palace on the Water (Royal Baths Museum), Warsaw. While living in Turkey between 1716 and 1718, Lady Mary Wortley Montagu learned about the use of variolation to inoculate against smallpox. On her return to England she became a staunch promoter of the practice. *(Wikimedia Commons)*

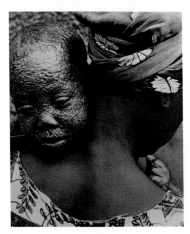

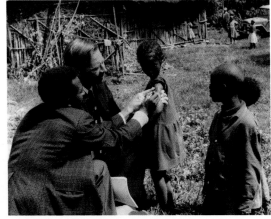

A todlder with smallpox in the Democratic Republic of the Congo, 1970s. *(Wellcome Collection: CC BY)*

DA Henderson (second left), head of the WHO's Intensive Smallpox Eradication Programme, visiting a vaccination clinic in Ethiopia in the 1970s. *(Alamy)*

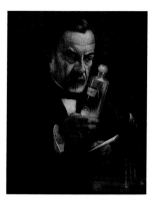

Louis Pasteur at work in his laboratory (left) and in the field (right), inoculating sheep against anthrax in a field trial at Pouilly-le-Fort, France, 1881. *(Both Wellcome Collection CC BY)*

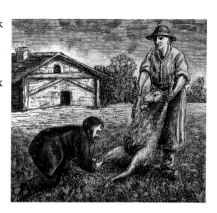

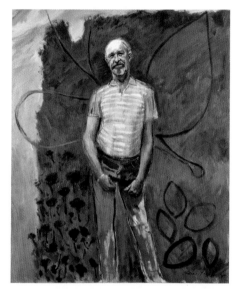

Flugelman with Wingman, Guy Warren's 1985 Archibald Prize–winning portrait of fellow artist Bert Flugelman, who bravely battled polio. *(Courtesy of Guy Warren/Art Gallery of New South Wales)*

Spanish artist Joaquín Sorolla's 1899 painting *Sad Inheritance* shows a monk helping two youngsters affected by polio to bathe in the sea near Valencia with other children. A polio epidemic had struck the city some years earlier. *(Wikimedia Commons)*

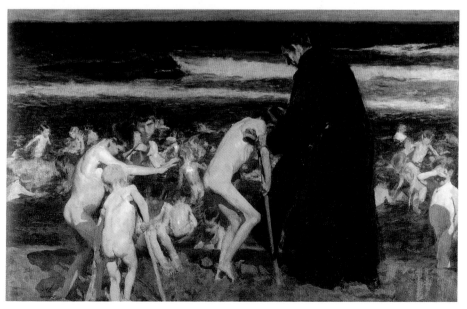

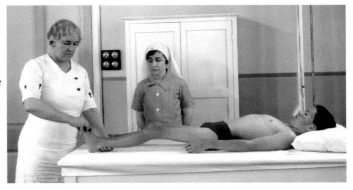

Australian nurse Sister Elizabeth Kenny (at left) won international fame for her unconventional polio treatments. *(State Library of Queensland)*

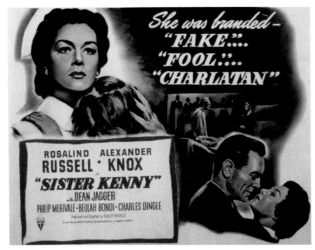

Such was Sister Kenny's popularity in the United States that a Hollywood movie was made about her in 1946. The glamorous Rosalind Russell played Sister Kenny. *(Alamy)*

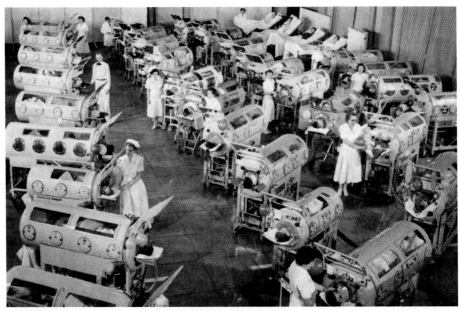

Polio patients in iron lungs, Rancho Los Amigos Respirator Center, California, 1953. Most recovered within days but some remained in an iron lung for the rest of their lives. *(Alamy)*

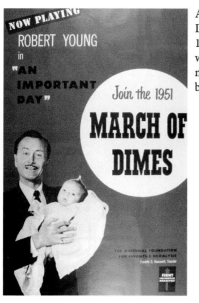

Actor Robert Young helped promote the March of Dimes campaign for polio prevention. Founded in 1938 by President Franklin Roosevelt, who himself was a victim of the disease, the March of Dimes did much to raise awareness in the United States of the benefits of immunisation. *(Alamy)*

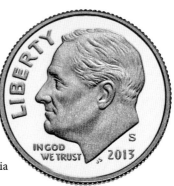

In 1946 a special dime was issued to commemorate Roosevelt's efforts to fight polio. (Wikimedia Commons)

Scientists Jonas Salk (right) and Albert Sabin (far right) developed different polio vaccines in the 1950s and competed with each other for the rest of their lives. Between them, they saved millions from dying of or being crippled by polio. *(Wikimedia Commons/Alamy)*

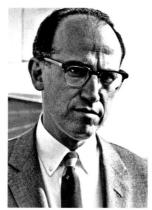

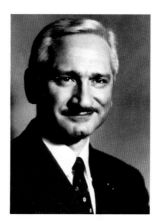

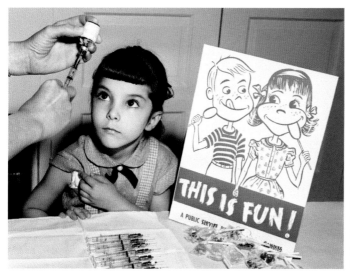

Cartoons and candies sweetened the deal for younger children during the 1950s United States polio vaccination campaign, though this young lady does not look convinced the jab won't hurt. *(Alamy)*

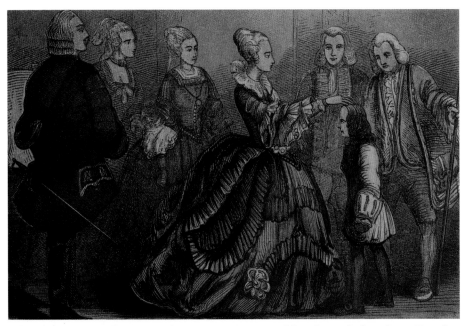

A 'royal touch' was said to protect the recipient against scrofula, a form of tuberculosis. Here the young Samuel Johnson, later a distinguished literary figure, receives this somewhat unreliable protection from Queen Anne in London in 1712. *(Alamy)*

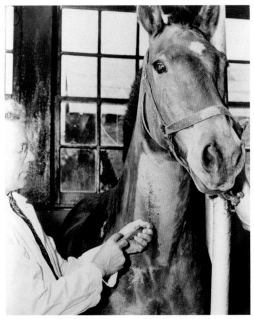

In the early 1900s, researchers found that injecting diphtheria toxin into a horse caused the animal to produce antibodies. In turn the antibodies could be used to create an antitoxin that would protect humans from the disease. *(Library of Congress)*

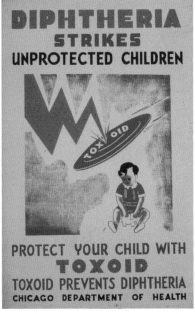

DIPHTHERIA STRIKES UNPROTECTED CHILDREN

TOXOID

PROTECT YOUR CHILD WITH TOXOID

TOXOID PREVENTS DIPHTHERIA

CHICAGO DEPARTMENT OF HEALTH

By the early 1930s, a vaccine based on a toxoid – a toxin weakened with heat and drugs – had replaced diphtheria antitoxin as the most effective treatment. *(Library of Congress)*

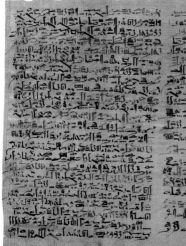

The Edwin Smith Papyrus, an Egyptian document dating from 1600 BC – and possibly much earlier – contains the first known description of the symptoms of tetanus. *(Wikimedia Commons)*

An infant aged 11 months being ventilated for measles pneumonia. He eventually recovered from this life-threatening illness. Though often regarded as a mild disease, measles is in fact a killer. Before the advent of a vaccine, 2.6 million children worldwide died of the disease every year. *(David Isaacs)*

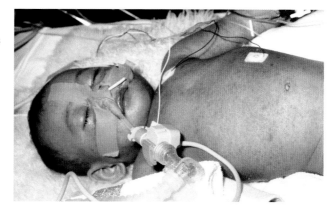

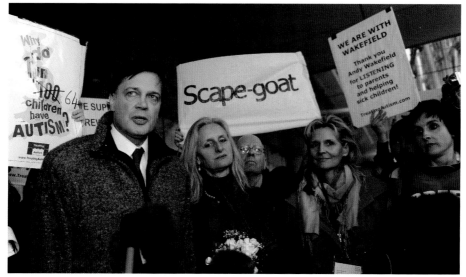

Anti-vaccination campaigner Andrew Wakefield, flanked by his supporters, gives a statement to the press outside the General Medical Council headquarters in London in 2010. *(Alamy)*

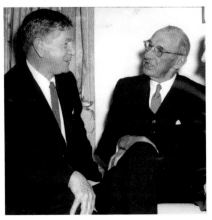

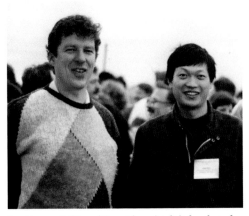

Great Australians: scientist and Nobel laureate Sir Macfarlane Burnet (left) meets Sir Norman Gregg, the ophthalmologist who first described babies with congenital rubella syndrome. *(State Library of Victoria)*

Ian Frazer (left) and Jian Zhou (right) developed the world's first human papillomavirus vaccine at the University of Queensland. In countries where the vaccine has been administered widely, the incidence of cervical cancer has fallen dramatically. *(Courtesy of Ian Frazer)*

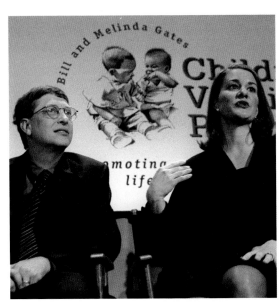

Bill and Melinda Gates in 1998 at the launch of the Children's Vaccine Program, which led in turn to the creation of Gavi, the Vaccine Alliance. Today, millions of children owe their lives to immunisations delivered by Gavi. *(Getty Images)*

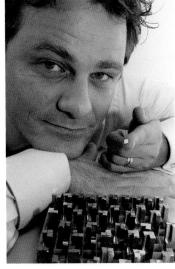

Professor Mark Kendall of the University of Queensland displaying his 'nanopatch'. This tiny patch covered in microscopic needles efficiently and painlessly delivers a vaccine to the abundant immune cells just under the skin. *(Courtesy of Mark Kendall)*

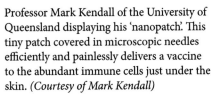

The highest incidence of pneumococcal infection is in infants, who can get meningitis as well as pneumonia, and in the elderly, who tend just to get pneumonia. Pneumococcal pneumonia can be treated with antibiotics, but has a high mortality rate in the elderly.

There are two major types of vaccine against pneumococcal infection. Pneumococcal polysaccharide vaccine (PPV) was first developed in 1945, and is made from the bacteria's purified sugar coating. (Polysaccharide is a scientific name for sugar.) The most commonly used vaccine contains 23 different sugars from 23 different strains of pneumococcus and is sometimes called 23v-PPV (23-valent pneumococcal polysaccharide vaccine). This vaccine certainly works reasonably well in young and middle-aged adults, but its effectiveness in the elderly is controversial.

Polysaccharide vaccines are now being replaced by conjugate vaccines in which the polysaccharide sugar capsules are conjugated (chemically joined) to proteins. This technique has been important for developing vaccines against three organisms that can cause meningitis in babies: pneumococcus, meningococcus and Hib. The same conjugate pneumococcal vaccines that work well in infancy also work well in old age. They are more expensive than polysaccharide vaccines, but prices can often be negotiated. Some countries such as Australia and the United States have changed from pneumococcal polysaccharide (PPV) to pneumococcal conjugate vaccines (PCV) for the elderly, and other countries are highly likely to follow suit.

Pneumococcal conjugate vaccine had been introduced in 134 countries by the end of 2016; the WHO estimated that global coverage in 2016 was 42%.

Tetanus

Elderly adults occasionally develop tetanus from a dirty wound – often, if they are keen gardeners, a rose-thorn prick contaminated by soil containing manure. Antibody levels tend to fall with time after immunisation, but those with low levels who have been immunised have 'immune memory' that can boost their antibodies.

Tetanus is rare in well-immunised populations. However, some elderly people have never been immunised, and many of them do not know it. For this reason, booster immunisations that include tetanus (usually diphtheria-tetanus-pertussis vaccine) are recommended for the elderly in many countries every 10 years.

Maintaining immunity

Our immune system is weakest and we are most susceptible to infections at the extremes of life. Immunisation reduces the likelihood that the elderly will catch life-threatening infections like influenza and pneumococcal pneumonia, or fall prey to debilitating shingles.

As French singer Maurice Chevalier said: 'Old age isn't so bad when you consider the alternative.' But good health in old age is a whole lot better than bad health, particularly if the bad health could easily have been prevented by immunisation.

CHAPTER 11

The tragedies and the frauds

The history of immunisation has been punctuated by tragedies and the victims have mainly been children. Some tragedies came about as scientists and researchers wrestled with technology, or struggled to understand the complexity of the human immune response. Some occurred because of well-meaning but ill-founded fears about vaccine safety. And at least one came about because of fraud.

Early tragedies in the United States

As we learned in Chapter 6, the German physiologist Emil von Behring proved that horse serum containing diphtheria antitoxin could help infected children recover from diphtheria. He later showed that tetanus antitoxin horse serum could protect war-wounded men against tetanus. For these discoveries he was awarded the Nobel Prize in 1901. Ironically, it was in that very year that the first major vaccine tragedy – relating to the same two diseases – occurred.

On 19 October, a St Louis physician, Dr RC Harris, was called to the home of Bessie Baker, a young girl who had diphtheria. He gave her an injection of diphtheria antitoxin and told her parents she would soon be entirely well. He also injected her two younger siblings with antitoxin to protect them from developing diphtheria.

Four days later he returned to the house. In an interview in the *St Louis Post Dispatch*, Dr Harris was quoted as saying: 'There I found that the little girl was suffering from tetanus (lockjaw). I could do nothing for her. The poison was injected so thoroughly into her system that she was beyond medical aid.' The spasms of her face and throat muscles would have been agonising. Within a week her two siblings also died from tetanus.

The antitoxin Dr Harris had given to the three children had been made by injecting diphtheria toxin into a retired milk-wagon horse called Jim. Jim had produced about 30 litres of antitoxin in three years, which had saved many children's lives. But alas, Jim had contracted tetanus and had had to be put down. Horses can catch tetanus through infected cuts or, as is most likely in Jim's case, through eating contaminated soil or droppings. Some serum taken from Jim two days before he was destroyed should have been discarded, but had unwisely been used to make the diphtheria antitoxin that killed the three Baker children and 10 other children in St Louis who were given the same antitoxin.

That same year, nine children in Camden, New Jersey, died after being given smallpox vaccine also contaminated with tetanus.

At this time vaccines were often manufactured privately in the United States, with little supervision of the way the serum was produced. The next year, 1902, the United States passed the *Biologics Control Act*, which regulated vaccine and antitoxin production, required manufacturers to be licensed and mandated regular inspections of manufacturing facilities. Vaccine quality and safety improved, although, as we will see, the new procedures were not infallible.

The Lübeck tragedy

These American cautionary tales were not heeded sufficiently elsewhere. BCG vaccine to protect against tuberculosis was first made in France in 1921. In December 1929, the Lübeck General Hospital in northern Germany started to offer BCG vaccine to newborn babies, to reduce the risk of catching TB. Vials of BCG vaccine were shaken and some vaccine was added to a spoon of warm breast milk and given to the babies to drink.

Tragically, some vaccine vials were inadvertently contaminated with live *Mycobacterium tuberculosis* from the laboratory where the BCG was prepared. Over the next four months, 251 newborn babies were fed contaminated vaccine. While older children and adults usually develop no symptoms when infected with TB, newborns are more susceptible. Before they were three months old, babies delivered at the hospital were starting to die at a much higher rate than expected. Within a year, 90% of babies given the contaminated vaccine had developed clinical or X-ray evidence of TB, mostly in the lymph nodes, and 72 babies had died.

The Lübeck accident was global news, and a setback to acceptance of immunisation in general and BCG vaccine in particular. To this day, the United States and the Netherlands have never routinely immunised children with BCG.

The Bundaberg tragedy

Bundaberg is a small city in sugar-cane country four hours' drive north of Brisbane, at the southern tip of the Great Barrier Reef. Bundaberg is famous for its rum, and infamous for an early vaccine disaster.

In the 1920s, diphtheria was a major problem in Bundaberg; during 1926 and 1927 more than 200 locals were infected with the disease and three died. An immunisation program was started in January 1928. On the 10th day of the program, 21 children aged 23 months to seven years were given the vaccine. Within hours, 18 of them became desperately ill. On 30 January 1928, the *Bundaberg Daily News and Mail* reported:

> Begun on January 17, the inoculation went apparently well until Friday night when children who were given injections that day showed alarming symptoms. These developed rapidly to virulent and fatal blood poisoning resembling anthrax. Twelve children on Saturday died despite all efforts to save them and several more are in critical and dangerous states.
>
> Consternation prevails ... Last night the Mayor set in train with the Authorities concerned proposals to the Education Department to allow state school children to parade to-day as a tribute to their dead comrades.
>
> It is an old but true saying 'in the midst of life we are in death'. Today Bundaberg mourns the loss of twelve fine little

children, whose bright young lives were nipped in the bud, as the result of some maleficent quality that developed or was hidden in the immunising serum injected into their arms on Friday for the purpose of assuring their safety against the dreaded diphtheria that is so threatening at this time.

The victims are:–

Thomas Robinson, 5½ years

William Robinson, 4 years

Mervyn Robinson, 23 months

Edward Baker, 5 years

Keith Baker, 3 years

George Baker, 6 years

Marsden Coates, 7 years

William Follitt, 2½ years

Mary Sheppard, 5 years

Monica Sheppard, 2½ years

Myrtle Brennan, 3½ years

Joan Peterson, 5½ years

One family lost all three of their sons, and one of the city councillors lost his two sons. The most likely cause was that the vaccine vial used for all the injections was accidentally contaminated with a toxin-producing strain of the *Staphylococcus aureus* bacterium ('golden staph'). The tragedy was considered a public health disaster in Australia and it attracted attention globally. A royal commission was set up to investigate the causes.

One positive outcome of the tragedy was that it taught authorities important safety lessons. The contamination probably occurred because of repeated puncturing of a rubber bung on a multi-dose vial. Multi-dose vaccine vials were not used again for many years. However, they were used without mishap to deliver influenza vaccine during the 2011 influenza pandemic, because of the need to give many doses in a very short time.

The Bundaberg vaccine was not refrigerated and the Queensland January heat probably contributed to the growth of the contaminating bacteria. The tragedy led to recognition of the importance of keeping vaccines refrigerated to maintain the 'cold chain'. Vaccines can still deteriorate if left unrefrigerated all day, and the problems can be compounded if the same syringe is used to give multiple doses, as happened in a remote village in South Sudan in 2017, when 15 children died from contaminated vaccine during a poorly conducted measles immunisation program. The program nevertheless ended a measles epidemic and saved hundreds of lives.

The Bundaberg vaccine also did not contain any preservatives or antiseptics to prevent contamination. Almost all vaccines now contain small amounts of disinfectants, such as phenol or phenoxyethanol, to prevent contamination with bacteria or fungi. The evidence suggests that these are not harmful and perform an essential role in maintaining sterility.

From time to time concerns have been raised about preservatives, particularly thiomersal (sometimes called thimerosal), which contains minuscule amounts of mercury and was once used commonly in vaccines. Although there is less mercury in any vaccine than we consume when eating fish, it is very difficult to prove scientifically that something is definitely not harmful. The United States Institute of Medicine reported in 2001 that there was insufficient evidence to prove or disprove whether thiomersal causes autism, attention deficit hypersensitivity disorder, or speech or language delay. In 2004 the institute reported that the evidence now favours 'rejection of a causal relationship between thimerosal-containing vaccines and autism'.

When, in the late 1990s, fears of possible harm from mercury poisoning were raised in Europe and North America, the response of most affluent countries was to try to reassure the public that thiomersal was safe, while instituting measures to remove it from most vaccines or reduce its concentration considerably. This sort of mixed message – 'Thiomersal is safe, but we'll remove it just to be sure' – is at best confusing and at worst bad for public confidence in vaccine safety. Some experts who were convinced there was firm evidence that thiomersal was not harmful felt it would have been better to try to reassure the public while not changing the vaccines.

Vaccines also contain non-toxic stabilising additives such as gelatin, lactose, sucrose, sorbitol and mannitol. Furthermore, as we have discussed, since the 1920s very small amounts of aluminium salts (alum) have been added to many vaccines as an adjuvant. The amount of aluminium in vaccines is minimal; there is more in most normal foods and far more in antacids. Adjuvants are only used when vaccines do not stimulate an adequate immune response without them.

Concerns about alum arose when studies suggested a possible link between chronic aluminium exposure and Alzheimer's disease. Though this link remains controversial and unproved, papers continue to be published in journals questioning the safety of aluminium in vaccines. In 2004, Tom Jefferson, an American expert on vaccine safety and efficacy, reviewed five studies involving a total of over 12,000 infants and children, comparing DTP vaccines containing aluminium with those containing no aluminium. He found no evidence that aluminium salts in vaccines cause any serious or long-lasting adverse events.

Clearly, we need to be sure that any new adjuvants we use are safe. We can only know this by studying the effects of vaccines containing them. If the vaccines prove safe, the adjuvants must be too. There will always be theoretical concerns that adverse effects may not emerge for many years, but similar concerns apply to many products we use, including foods.

There is a saying 'to pour oil on troubled waters'. Oil and water do not mix. In the body too, oily substances like lipids repel water, yet we would like to deliver vaccines to all parts of the body. Many of the new adjuvants we use have been designed to deliver the vaccines to remote sites. Liposome adjuvants are small round particles comprising a drop of liquid enclosed in one or more layers of lipid – effectively a water droplet enclosed in fat. Water-soluble proteins can be trapped in the liquid centre and protected by the fat layer until they reach the desired target site. The adjuvant AS01, used in a malaria vaccine given to children in clinical trials, is liposome-based.

Oil-in-water emulsions can also be used as adjuvants. An example is MF-59. The adjuvanted influenza vaccine introduced in 2018 in Australia to give better protection to the elderly contains MF-59.

The oil most commonly used in oil-in-water adjuvants is squalene oil, a naturally occurring oily compound. Shark-liver oil was the original source of squalene, but squalene oils can also be sourced from various plants.

Some new adjuvants are saponins, soapy substances that can make cell membranes leaky and allow proteins to penetrate. Saponins are also naturally occurring substances found mainly in plants; they can be sourced from sea cucumbers.

Studies of over 25,000 children exposed to vaccines containing one of four new adjuvants – AS01, AS02, AS03 and MF59 – showed they were significantly less likely to experience immediate serious side effects than children receiving conventional vaccines. Although the long-term adverse effects still need to be monitored, these results are encouraging.

The yellow fever vaccine

A cynical view might be that the Western world only gets interested in diseases of third-world countries when they affect war or trade or both. Yellow fever is a disease of developing countries in West Africa and Central and South America, but a vaccine only came about when the United States wanted to protect workers building the Panama Canal around 1900. Sadly, this vaccine has had a chequered history, both before and since its development.

Yellow fever virus infects and inflames the liver, causing hepatitis and jaundice. Jaundice is yellow discolouration of the skin caused by build-up in the bloodstream of a pigment, bilirubin, a breakdown product of blood cells normally cleared by the liver. The name 'yellow fever' derives from this jaundice. The virus is transmitted to humans by mosquitoes that have bitten other infected humans or monkeys. It is another example of a human infection that originated in animals – in this case monkeys. Most Westerners only know about it because they have to get yellow fever vaccine to travel to Africa or South America, but it has been and remains a major killer in those areas. In 2013, the WHO estimated there were 84,000 to 170,000 severe cases of yellow fever and 29,000 to 60,000 deaths worldwide, of which 90% were in Africa.

Yellow fever started in Africa and spread to Central and South America with the slave trade. It became particularly important to the Western world because of the disruption it caused to trade, and was sometimes called 'yellow jack' after the yellow quarantine flag hoisted by affected ships.

Yellow fever even spread to the United States, causing an outbreak in New York in 1668, and one in Philadelphia in 1793, which killed 9% of the city's population. George Washington's government was based in Philadelphia and he and it fled the city. Yellow fever also spread to Spain in the 19th century, causing outbreaks in Gibraltar and Barcelona, which killed thousands.

In the late 1800s Western powers came up with the idea of cutting an artificial canal across the narrow Isthmus of Panama in Central America to provide a maritime trade waterway between the Atlantic and Pacific Oceans, allowing ships to bypass treacherous Cape Horn on the southern tip of South America. The French started building the Panama Canal in 1881 but abandoned the project. This was due partly to engineering problems – but mainly to worker deaths from tropical diseases, particularly yellow fever and malaria.

In 1902 the American government of Theodore Roosevelt passed the 'Spooner Act' (Senator Spooner wrote the Act) which paid the French a large sum to take over building the Panama Canal. Knowing the problems the French had faced, the United States military had appointed a commission in 1900, headed by army doctor and yellow fever specialist Walter Reed, to investigate the cause of yellow fever and how to prevent it.

A British doctor, Ronald Ross, working in India, had shown in 1896 that malaria was transmitted through mosquito bites. Reed's team performed experiments that established that yellow fever is also transmitted by infected mosquitoes. These studies led the American military to literally pour oil on the troubled Panama waterways to prevent mosquitoes from breeding, and to apply larvicides if they did. This successfully prevented most of the yellow fever in Panama.

But the research was not without its failures. Although Reed was reasonably cautious, three United States army volunteers died from being injected with small doses of yellow fever.

One promising researcher on Reed's team, 34-year-old Dr Jesse Lazear, wrote a letter to his wife in September 1900: 'I rather think I am on the track of the real germ.' Unfortunately the germ was on *his* track. Two and a half weeks later, Dr Lazear died from yellow fever. He had allowed an infected mosquito to bite him in an attempt to prove that mosquitoes transmitted the disease. The military covered up the fact that Dr Lazear had infected himself deliberately, and the truth was only discovered in 1947 from Dr Lazear's own notebook.

The tragedies connected with yellow fever did not end in Panama. In the 1930s a live attenuated virus vaccine against yellow fever was developed. It soon became the third most widely used human vaccine after the smallpox and rabies vaccines. During World War II, fighting in yellow-fever-endemic zones such as North Africa led to a huge demand for yellow fever vaccine. Over 15 months from 1941 to 1942, the United States Army immunised 7 million troops. However, the vaccine had been stabilised with human serum, and one of the serum donors had had chronic hepatitis B infection. A little hepatitis B goes a long way: the entire supply of yellow fever vaccine was contaminated with hepatitis B virus. This led to many thousands of cases of hepatitis B, and an estimated 100 deaths. The *Chicago*

Tribune sourly pointed out that 20 times as many soldiers had fallen victim to the vaccine in North Africa as had been wounded in battle.

Today the vaccine is safe and is given to travellers to countries where yellow fever is endemic, and the WHO is increasingly using it to prevent the disease. Between 2005 and 2016, over 105 million people were vaccinated across 14 of 34 endemic African countries.

The Cutter Incident

We heard in Chapter 4 about the race to develop a polio vaccine, and the fierce rivalry between two brilliant men, virologists Albert Sabin and Jonas Salk. Salk's killed (inactivated) polio vaccine (IPV) was first off the blocks, ready to be tested in a large randomised controlled trial by 1954.

The American public, petrified of a disease that could infect thousands of children in a few days, was so desperate that compromises were being made even before the trial results were announced.

Jonas Salk had struggled to prepare enough safe vaccine in which all the poliovirus was definitely killed and which stimulated an immune response when injected. Salk could not make industrial quantities of IPV himself, so pharmaceutical companies were encouraged to apply for licences to make the vaccine, the understanding being that they were almost certain to get them. One of these companies, Eli Lilly, paid US$250,000 (equivalent to US$2 million now) to broadcast the announcement of the trial results on closed-circuit television to cinemas across the land. No conflict of interest there, then.

At 2.45pm, just three hours after the announcement of the trial findings, a licensing committee met to consider applications to manufacture IPV from five pharmaceutical companies: Eli Lilly, Parke-Davis, Pitman-Moore, Wyeth and Cutter Laboratories. The committee was looking for the first time at applications that nowadays would take a year to approve. They were a little pressed for time, because the United States Secretary of Health had arranged a press conference for 4.15pm that day, when she would publicly sign the licences. No pressure.

All five companies were granted licences and cardboard boxes of vaccines were shipped to health clinics the same evening. The speed of all this was breathtaking. But not all vaccines are created equal (with apologies to George Orwell for so mangling his wonderful line from *Animal Farm*).

All five companies had different methods of preparing the vaccine. There were safeguards: each company had to prove to the national Laboratory of Biologics Control that it had made 11 consecutive batches of IPV that contained no live poliovirus. However, these stringent requirements were relaxed as the intended vaccine launch approached, and companies were not required to document their failures along the way.

Bernice Eddy from the Laboratory of Biologics Control tested a preliminary IPV vaccine submitted by California-based family firm Cutter Laboratories. She inoculated the vaccine into the brains of 12 anaesthetised monkeys and into the muscles of another six. Half the batches Cutter submitted caused paralysis in the monkeys. There must have been live virus in the vaccine to give the monkeys polio. Although these batches of vaccine were never given to the public, Eddy feared Cutter Laboratories was using a flawed process. 'There's going to be a disaster. I know it,' she confided to a friend. She told her boss, but he did not inform the licensing committee.

Two weeks after the launch of the new vaccine, disaster struck. A contemporary scientific report detailed: 'On April 25, 1955, an infant with paralytic poliomyelitis was admitted to Michael Reese Hospital, Chicago, Illinois. The patient had been inoculated in the buttock ... on April 16, and developed flaccid paralysis of both legs on April 24.' Within days, the problem had been traced to the Cutter vaccine.

More than 200,000 children in the Western and Midwestern United States had been given Cutter's faulty vaccine, in which the live virus had not been killed. Of these, some 40,000 children developed polio, 200 were paralysed permanently and 10 died. Cutter promptly withdrew its vaccine.

The Cutter Incident (as it came to be called) was a major catastrophe. American immunisation expert Paul Offit has discussed its origins in great detail in his fascinating book *The Cutter Incident*. In 1998 and 1999, Offit spoke at length to Julius Youngner, who was a young member of Salk's laboratory staff at the time of the incident.

The day after the contracts were signed, Youngner was rung by the Associate Director of Research at Cutter Laboratories to say they were having trouble inactivating poliovirus for their vaccine and the live virus was persisting for days. Youngner immediately visited their manufacturing plant in Berkeley, California. He was appalled to find an amateurish setup and had serious concerns about their ability to reliably inactivate live poliovirus. He later told Offit: 'They looked like they didn't know what the Hell they were doing.' When he returned to Philadelphia, Youngner told Salk about his concerns and offered to write to the head of the

Laboratory of Biologics Control. Salk said he would write, but never did.

This is Youngner's memory of what happened, related over 40 years after the event. Salk is not alive to give his version, and the relationship between the two men after the Cutter Incident was far from cordial. However, Cutter Laboratories would not by any means be the last pharmaceutical company to cover up knowledge of safety concerns and risk lives in favour of profit.

Ben Goldacre is an Oxford doctor, academic and author. In his powerful book *Bad Pharma: How Drug Companies Mislead Doctors and Harm Patients*, he describes the lengths to which some pharmaceutical companies will go to promote drugs they know are not only ineffective but frankly harmful. It is little wonder that vaccine sceptics are suspicious of the motives of vaccine companies, although improved safeguards make it incredibly unlikely we will ever have another Cutter Incident.

The small family firm of Cutter Laboratories was clearly culpable. Its vaccine was associated with far, far more cases of paralysis than the vaccines made by any of the four other well-established pharmaceutical companies. Three of these companies' vaccines had not caused any increase in paralysis at all. But one batch of Wyeth vaccine was associated with considerably more cases of paralysis than any of Wyeth's other batches. Did Wyeth immunise children with one vaccine batch that contained live virus? The figures were suggestive but not definitive. It might have been pure chance. For example, the children who received the suspect batch might have been coming down with polio already. The suspect batch was quietly removed from the shelves and the public was not informed. In late 1955 Neal Nathanson who worked at the Centers for Disease Control (CDC) coauthored a report called *The Wyeth Problem*, in which he raised his suspicion that children were indeed given a batch of Wyeth vaccine which inadvertently contained live poliovirus, although he does not mention a cover-up. Nathanson wrote many scientific papers about the Cutter Incident, but never published a paper expressing any concerns about the Wyeth vaccine. History does not relate whether he was advised by his superiors at the CDC, a federal public health agency, not to publish any further details for fear of worrying the public about the continuing IPV program. There was to be no Wyeth Incident. Was this a cover-up or a wise precautionary measure to allay public concern?

There was a government inquiry into the Cutter Incident, of course. A congressional hearing heard witnesses blame FDR's National Foundation for Infantile Paralysis, which funded the trial; the Laboratory of Biologics Control, which controlled vaccine safety; and Jonas Salk, who they alleged had developed a faulty technique for killing the vaccine virus. Many people working in vaccine regulation were sacked, from the most senior to the most junior.

Politicians blamed politicians. Senator Wayne Morse of Oregon said: 'The federal government inspects meat in the slaughterhouse more carefully than it has inspected the polio vaccine.' Some tried to blame then Vice President Richard Nixon for purportedly putting pressure on authorities to license the vaccine. He didn't. Nixon might have been responsible for Watergate, but he didn't cause the Cutter Incident.

Cutter Laboratories never admitted it was at fault. It said the problem was a general one that applied to all IPV, even though Cutter vaccines caused many more cases of paralysis than any of the other companies' vaccines, including Wyeth's. Mostly Cutter

Laboratories blamed the government for inadequate testing. Walter Ward, the scientist who led Cutter's IPV development program, asserted that Jonas Salk's technique for killing the virus was the only cause of the disaster, which Ward always referred to as 'the Salk Incident'.

Several leading scientists, including Salk's lifelong rival Albert Sabin and Nobel Prize laureate John Enders, advised Congress and the assembled media throng to stop the IPV immunisation program. During a less public government meeting, Enders told Salk pointedly: 'It is quack medicine to pretend that this is a killed vaccine when you know that it has live virus in it. Every batch has live virus in it.' The usually sanguine Salk was shaken. He later said he felt suicidal for the first time in his life.

But the United States Government, and indeed the public, had too much invested in the polio prevention program to stop now. The IPV immunisation program continued. Initially uptake was patchy. The American public was understandably confused by the mixed messages: the government and the vaccine companies were saying IPV was safe, whereas leading United States scientists including a Nobel Prize winner said it was not.

In a timely but tragic twist of fate, less than three months after the Cutter vaccine was withdrawn, the United States was hit by a nationwide polio epidemic. More than 1700 people were paralysed. There was no randomised control trial in place, but the outbreak provided ample evidence of vaccine efficacy. The rate of polio in unimmunised people was 20 per 1000. The rate in people who had received one dose of IPV was 10 in 1000, half as much. The rate after two doses was 5 per 1000, a quarter as much. The rate after the ideally recommended three doses was zero. That is why we now give three doses of polio vaccine.

One positive was that the Cutter Incident led to highly effective federal regulation of vaccine production. Regulations on vaccine safety were tightened, and the number of vaccine regulatory staff was increased from 10 in 1955 to 150 by 1956. The United States has had an incomparably unblemished safety record ever since. Vaccine regulation was moved to the United States Food and Drug Administration in 1972, which now has more than 250 staff dealing solely with vaccine safety. Because they are given to everyone, vaccines need to be even safer than pharmaceuticals, and indeed they now are.

In the longer term, the Cutter Incident did not have a lasting adverse effect on the uptake of polio vaccine in the United States or elsewhere. Polio was and is a truly terrible disease, and almost everyone in the 1950s and 1960s knew a family who had a paralysed child. Most people were prepared to accept that the Cutter Incident was an isolated accident, and that the Salk vaccine was subsequently made safe. Memory of infectious diseases, and particularly visible evidence of their ravages, are powerful drivers of vaccine acceptance.

The Cutter Incident had another less beneficial outcome, however. Cutter Laboratories was sued by the parents of a child with severe permanent paralysis, and this case acted as a test case for 60 other suits. In a confusing jury trial, it was found that Cutter Laboratories had not been negligent, but the company was still ordered to pay compensation to those injured by the vaccine. This was, without precedent, liability without fault. Americans have a long history of suing for anything and everything, but this was the start of a new saga. A pharmaceutical company could be sued successfully, despite following the regulations, if someone given a vaccine developed a rare, known side effect, even if they had been warned about it. The verdict precipitated a climate of litigation against vaccine companies, which had a detrimental effect on vaccine production.

You don't need to feel too sorry for Cutter Laboratories, though. The company paid the compensation and thrived, making pharmaceuticals as well as vaccines. By 1962 it had assets of over US$18 million, 80% more than in 1955. In 1978 it was bought by the German pharmaceutical company Bayer.

The losers were the children who developed polio, not Cutter.

The MMR–autism controversy

The United Kingdom whole-cell pertussis vaccine controversy in the 1970s, described in Chapter 1, was soon proved spectacularly and tragically wrong when whooping cough returned to the United Kingdom with a vengeance between 1977 and 1979. Even though concerns that the vaccine could cause brain damage proved unfounded, it is unlikely that the public was ever totally reassured.

This was fertile ground for another vaccine controversy, and one with even greater repercussions: the claim that there was a possible link between measles-mumps-rubella (MMR) vaccine and autism. The controversy started at the Royal Free Hospital in the London suburb of Hampstead, a major teaching hospital with a proud history. (I have personal links: I grew up in Hampstead, my eldest son, Ben, was born at the Royal Free, and a dear friend was until recently a consultant neurologist there. What is more, John Keats wrote 'Ode to a Nightingale' just down the hill from the Royal Free.)

When Andrew Wakefield came to work at the Royal Free Hospital as a consultant gastroenterologist in 1997, research there was in the doldrums. Wakefield arrived like a breath of fresh air. He was eloquent, with an infectious enthusiasm. He persuaded colleagues to join him in research that he said was at the cutting edge, and promised them their work would be published in high-powered journals. There were even whispers of a Nobel Prize. Wakefield had long been interested in a possible link between inflammatory diseases of the bowel, such as Crohn's disease, and measles virus infection. In 1993, he had published research suggesting measles virus might cause Crohn's disease and in 1995 a paper suggesting a link between measles vaccine and Crohn's disease. These findings excited interest but could not be replicated by other researchers.

A year after he started at the Royal Free, Wakefield and his colleagues submitted a paper based on 12 children with autism whom they said had been referred consecutively (one after the other) to the gastroenterology department because of gut symptoms (diarrhoea, abdominal pain, bloating, food intolerance). The authors claimed that 8 of these 12 children displayed symptoms of autism soon after they were given MMR vaccine and one displayed symptoms soon after catching measles infection.

It was 1998. The day the paper was published in the prestigious British journal *The Lancet*, 41-year-old Wakefield transfixed a packed press conference with a startling video news release. He claimed to have found the cause of autism: MMR vaccine. He said he had discovered a new 'bowel and brain' syndrome. He proposed that the MMR vaccine virus travelled in the bloodstream to the muscle supplying the gut, where it could grow and cause inflammation. The inflammation could allow unidentified, harmful proteins to enter the bloodstream and travel to the brain, causing autism. At this stage, he had no evidence to support his theory, but he was sure he would find it. Wakefield was articulate and charismatic; his claims made headline news.

Wakefield's assertion that MMR vaccine caused autism was outrageously bad science. The Royal Free team only studied 12 children already known to have autism. Their claim that eight of the children experienced a sudden onset of autism after MMR vaccine was puzzling, as autism is a chronic condition and had not previously been associated with a specific trauma. When trying to prove that a trauma actually causes a disease, it is essential that a study includes a control group, in case the association between the supposed trauma (in this case MMR vaccine) and the disease (autism) is just a chance association (in which case the disease would occur equally commonly in the control group). Wakefield and his colleagues had no control group for comparison.

Yet in the summary of their *Lancet* article the authors wrote: 'We identified associated gastrointestinal disease and developmental regression in a group of previously normal children, which was generally associated in time with possible environmental triggers.' 'Developmental regression' implies that the children's development went backwards, and the paper unequivocally stated that the children were previously normal. The suggested 'environmental triggers' were MMR vaccine in eight children and measles infection in one. The paper quoted the parents as saying their children were developing normally until they were given MMR vaccine, but then within two weeks of MMR the child's behaviour changed and they lost skills – for example, some stopped talking.

The claims about new bowel changes were also suspect. The authors claimed to have found bowel changes, to which they gave a new name, 'autistic enterocolitis'. (Enterocolitis means 'inflamed bowel'.) Experts would later throw doubt on the veracity of the bowel changes. Furthermore, to describe the changes, Wakefield and his fellow authors performed endoscopies on 8 of the 12 children. Such an endoscopy, which involves sedating the child and inserting a tube with a camera down the child's throat and into the bowel, is quite invasive. As many as three people were occasionally needed to hold a patient down to perform endoscopy. The ethics of performing such procedures on children was also later called into question.

Wakefield proposed that instead of MMR vaccine, children should be immunised with measles vaccine, mumps vaccine and rubella vaccine separately, with at least a year between each vaccination. In his press conference, Wakefield said: 'One more case of autism is too many. It's a moral issue for me and I can't support the continued use of these vaccines given in combination until this issue has been resolved.' How ironic and, indeed, cynical that Wakefield, who would prove to have falsified most of the data in the paper for personal financial gain, would claim this was a moral issue for him.

Wakefield said autism did not follow measles vaccine when it was given alone in 1968, but did follow MMR when it was given in 1988, but this ignored the fact that diagnostic criteria had changed enormously and children were diagnosed with autism far more often in 1988 than in 1968. There was no credible scientific rationale for Wakefield's claim that giving the same three vaccine viruses separately was safer than giving them combined in MMR vaccine.

In any case, measles, mumps and rubella vaccines were no longer made as separate vaccines in 1998. The effect of Wakefield's suggestion to split the vaccines was that the public had to choose between MMR and no vaccine at all. When British Prime Minister Tony Blair was asked if he had given MMR vaccine to his youngest child, who was due for vaccination, he refused to answer. Everyone took that as a no. The public was confused. Officials were warning them of the danger of measles and Wakefield was warning them of the danger of the vaccine. Who were they to believe?

The MMR–autism link excited global interest, and Wakefield travelled abroad spreading his message. In 2000, Wakefield talked at United States autism conferences and appeared on the CBS network's *60 Minutes* program saying that MMR was linked to what he called an 'epidemic of autism'. In 2003, more than five years after the *Lancet* paper, the United Kingdom's Channel 5 broadcast a 90-minute film called *Hear the Silence*. Hugh Bonneville played Andrew Wakefield and Juliet Stevenson played the mother of an autistic child. In the film, the mother cannot convince doctors that her child's autism started after the child was given MMR vaccine. But Dr Wakefield believes her. However, government officials decide they need to bring Wakefield down by portraying his research as flawed. They tap his phone and steal his files. But who is really behind Wakefield's persecution? In the film it is Big Pharma. The mother of another autistic child portrayed in the film says: 'It's a multi-million-pound industry, so they'll fight dirty.' The film got a modest television audience and decidedly mixed reviews, and was pilloried by outraged doctors. But its portrayal of the pharmaceutical industry and the government as the villains played right into the hands of the vaccine sceptics.

The *Lancet* paper was very bad science. But it took the persistence of one man, Brian Deer, to show that the research was fraudulent. Deer, an investigative journalist who specialised in inquiries into the pharmaceutical industry for the *Sunday Times*, was no respecter of reputations. He investigated Wakefield's paper from 2003 onwards, and his concerns about the ethics of the research grew and grew. He wrote a series of articles for the *Sunday Times* and also published papers in the *British Medical Journal (BMJ)*. He made a television documentary, *MMR: What They Didn't Tell You*, shown on Channel 4 in Britain in November 2004. Wakefield sued Deer for libel over the documentary, but subsequently dropped the case and was ordered to pay costs.

As Deer accumulated even more worrying data suggesting that the paper in *The Lancet* might contain serious errors of fact and that aspects of the research might have been unethical, the United Kingdom General Medical Council (GMC) decided to investigate the paper in detail. The GMC is the official body that oversees doctors' registration to practice. Wakefield and colleagues said it was unethical to investigate the 12 patients in the paper because it would infringe their privacy. But the GMC had the authority to look at the patients' case records. The GMC hearing against Wakefield commenced in July 2007. What the GMC uncovered over the following three years would leave its verdict in no doubt.

When you publish a scientific paper you must declare any potential conflicts of interest. Wakefield had declared to *The Lancet* that he had none, but in truth he had major financial conflicts. Wakefield had in fact been working for two years with a Norfolk solicitor, Richard Barr, on a lawsuit against the MMR vaccine companies, on behalf of parents who claimed the vaccine had been the cause of their child's autism. For this work, Wakefield was paid £150 (AU$265) an hour, and eventually earned a total of £435,643 (around AU$770,000) plus expenses. In addition, prior to the publication of his team's paper in *The Lancet*, Wakefield had lodged a patent for a new measles vaccine he called Transfer Factor, which he also claimed could be used to treat inflammatory bowel disease (he gave Transfer Factor to one of the research patients). If successful, his unscientific recommendation to give measles, mumps and rubella vaccines as separate vaccines instead of MMR could have made him a fortune.

The *Lancet* paper did not make it clear that the children had been selected by Wakefield rather than referred to the clinic for investigation in the normal way. At the time when Wakefield tested the children, many of their parents were already clients of Richard Barr, and Wakefield had found most of them through anti-MMR-vaccine campaign groups. Several parents had lodged compensation claims before the children were referred. None of the families lived in London. Two children were patients of the same doctor 450 kilometres from the Royal Free Hospital, three attended another clinic, and one was flown in from the United States.

Wakefield had declared to *The Lancet* that he had applied for and received Research Ethics Committee approval for the study, but he had misled the committee by claiming the children had been referred for treatment in the normal way. Arguably, Wakefield had used the 12 autistic children as guinea-pigs to prove a pre-formed theory. The *Lancet* paper claimed that all 12 children were previously normal, but the GMC found that five already had developmental problems before being given the MMR vaccine. Wakefield claimed that MMR vaccine had caused autism because the children had developed the condition within two weeks of receiving it, but it turned out that he had falsified data. The United States patient flown over specially to see Wakefield was reported in the *Lancet* paper as first developing symptoms of autism one week after receiving MMR vaccine, but the child's father insisted he had told Wakefield the symptoms had started two months before the child had been given the vaccine. Another patient was reported as becoming symptomatic two weeks after receiving MMR vaccine, yet the mother remembered it as being somewhere between two and six months afterwards. The facts did not fit with Wakefield's assertion of a close temporal relationship between vaccination and the onset of autistic symptoms, so Wakefield had simply changed the story to fit his theory.

On review by experts, the children's gut biopsies were found to be predominantly normal – certainly not nearly as abnormal as reported in the *Lancet* paper. Wakefield had changed diagnoses and histories to give the impression of a link between MMR, bowel disease and the sudden onset of autism that was not otherwise evident. Every one of the 12 cases had been altered substantially. As Brian Deer baldly stated: 'Wakefield had been secretly payrolled to create evidence against the [MMR] shot and, while planning extraordinary business schemes meant to profit from the scare, he had concealed, misreported and changed information about the children to rig the results published in the journal.'

This was high-stakes scientific fraud. None of Wakefield's 12 Royal Free co-authors had been aware of his deception, and all became increasingly alarmed as new revelations emerged. In 2004, as the full enormity of Wakefield's dubious research practices was starting to be uncovered by Brian Deer, *The Lancet* asked Wakefield and his co-authors to retract their paper. Ten retracted, including Professor John Walker-Smith and Dr Simon Murch, a junior consultant. Nevertheless, the GMC charged Walker-Smith and Murch, as well as Wakefield, with serious professional misconduct in 2004. Walker-Smith is a renowned Australian gastroenterologist who became Professor of Paediatric Gastroenterology at the University of London. I worked with him there. He had a picture of Queen Elizabeth II on his desk, flanked by miniature flags, a Union Jack and an Australian flag. He was always immaculately dressed, more English than the English, in eye-watering blue shirts with a starched white collar and a hospital tie. His middle initial is A, and his students and junior colleagues always referred to him as JAWS. Although we were at opposite ends of the political spectrum, I always admired John's intellectual integrity.

In the United States in 2009, the Federal Court heard a test case of petitions from some 5000 families that MMR vaccine had caused their children's autism. One of the presiding judges, George L Hastings, was highly sceptical of Wakefield's 'autistic enterocolitis', and said: 'Therefore, it is a noteworthy point that not only has that "autistic enterocolitis" theory not been accepted into gastroenterology textbooks, but that theory, and Dr Wakefield's role in its development, have been strongly criticized as constituting defective or fraudulent science.'

In 2010, a GMC panel of three doctors and two lay members found Wakefield guilty of dishonesty and of the abuse of developmentally challenged children, labelling him as 'unethical' and 'callous'. His research was found to be fraudulent and performed without valid ethical approval. The GMC struck Andrew Wakefield off the medical register. Wakefield was no longer allowed to be a medical doctor in the United Kingdom. In United States terms, this would be to revoke his licence to practice.

Five days later, *The Lancet* completely retracted the Wakefield paper from the scientific literature, declaring it was 'utterly false'.

It had been extraordinarily foolish, even negligent, of *The Lancet* to have published such poor science, and for the journal editors to have failed to recognise the damaging effect it might have. It had taken *The Lancet* 12 years to do the right thing.

In 2010, when the GMC found Andrew Wakefield guilty of research misconduct, it found John Walker-Smith guilty of the same charge and struck them both off the medical register. Simon Murch was exonerated. Professor Walker-Smith had retired nine years earlier. The GMC ruling seemed excessively punitive, since he was not party to Wakefield's fraud. In 2012, the High Court ruled that the GMC panel's decision about Professor Walker-Smith was flawed by 'inadequate and superficial reasoning' and overturned it. Andrew Wakefield argued that the High Court's decision vindicated him too, but his own application to the High Court to appeal the GMC ruling was turned down.

In 2011, the *BMJ* published damning papers by Brian Deer analysing the extent of Wakefield's research misdemeanours. Fiona Godlee, the *BMJ*'s editor-in-chief, wrote an accompanying editorial entitled 'Wakefield's Article Linking MMR Vaccine and Autism Was Fraudulent'. The same year, Brian Deer was awarded the British Press Award and the HealthWatch Award for his persistent and courageous investigation.

Wakefield denied everything, cried conspiracy and accused Deer and the *BMJ* of conducting a vendetta against him. Many United Kingdom doctors belong to a medical defence organisation, a form of doctor's insurance agency, which defends them if they are sued by a patient; Wakefield persuaded this organisation to embark on a lawsuit costing $2 million, which he abandoned after two years. His supporters still write on social media protesting his innocence.

The Royal Free Hospital offered Wakefield the opportunity to repeat his research, using a larger sample of 150 patients and with controls. The research never happened. Wakefield characteristically said his failure to take up the offer was the fault of others, rather than accepting that his bluff had been called and admitting he could not conduct the study, whose results he knew would be negative.

As a result of the controversy, measles immunisation rates fell markedly in the United Kingdom, from between 90 and 92% before the scandal to 80% in 2003 and as low as 30% in some areas. National rates did not reach 90% again until 2011. In the four years from 1998 to 2001, 10,794 cases of measles were reported nationally; between 2006 and 2009, that number rose to 17,654. We know that infectious diseases are under-reported, so the true impact of the Wakefield scandal on measles infection may have been much greater. About 1 in every 1000 children who catches measles will develop measles encephalitis; of every 10 children who develop measles encephalitis one will die, as Roald Dahl's daughter Olivia did, and two or three will have permanent brain damage. It is highly likely that the Wakefield scandal condemned many children to brain damage and left many others dead. For example, a small Dublin hospital admitted 11 children to hospital with measles in just seven months in the year 2000, and three of them died.

The controversy prompted a number of large scientific studies, all of which found no evidence whatsoever that MMR vaccine is a cause of autism. Ironically, the fall in MMR vaccine uptake in the United Kingdom provided a natural experiment: if Wakefield's claims were correct, rates of autism should have fallen too, but no such fall occurred.

The Wakefield MMR–autism saga is a sorry one for the medical profession and for the world, and the repercussions persist. Though MMR uptake in the United Kingdom has recovered to previously high levels, as we shall see in the next chapter, the MMR–autism debate has continued to resonate in Europe and the United States.

Vaccine surveillance and rotavirus

The many vaccine tragedies have not gone unheeded. Any new vaccine is extensively tested for efficacy and safety in clinical trials before it is introduced into the immunisation schedule. After it is introduced, intense post-marketing surveillance for adverse effects is conducted regionally and nationally in all industrialised and many developing countries. The aim of the surveillance is to detect extremely rare adverse effects, such as a one-in-a-million complication that could not be detected in clinical trials, even trials involving many thousands of subjects.

A good example of how contemporary surveillance works is what has happened with rotavirus vaccines. Immunisation with the first rotavirus vaccine, RotaShield, started in 1998 but was stopped in 1999 because surveillance showed that children given the vaccine had an increased risk of developing intussusception. This is a condition in which one section of the bowel telescopes into the next, which can prevent blood supply to the affected bowel. Intussusception is rare and can usually be corrected with medical or occasionally surgical treatment. Most cases occur in babies 5 to 10 months old, boys more often than girls. Some virus infections are associated with intussusception, presumably by causing damage or inflammation that affects the bowel.

Later rotavirus vaccines were studied on thousands of infants in randomised controlled trials, and the studies did not detect a significantly increased risk of intussusception. However, this did not mean it was certain that the new vaccines did *not* cause intussusception, only that the studies could not detect it; the increased risk was possibly too low for the studies to detect.

Surveillance studies showed that within three weeks of receiving their first and second doses of rotavirus vaccine babies did in fact have a slightly increased risk of developing intussusception. The risk was approximately six cases for every 100,000 infants vaccinated.

There is no doubt that in resource-poor countries the benefits of rotavirus vaccine far outweigh the relatively small number of extra cases of intussusception. Very few children die from rotavirus in wealthy countries, where the vaccine was introduced to reduce illness and hospitalisation rather than to save lives. In Australia, the vaccine prevents 7000 hospital admissions each year at the cost of 14 extra cases of intussusception. In the United States the equivalent figures are over 20,000 admissions prevented annually at the cost of about 50 extra cases of intussusception.

Thus rotavirus vaccines are not without some risk, but the public is informed of the risk and the health profession considers it acceptable.

Does money ever come into the equation in decisions about vaccine risk? Of course it does.

Health authorities in different countries had to choose whether to stay with OPV, knowing that 1 in every 2.5 million doses would paralyse a baby (about one baby every five years in Australia and eight babies a year in the United States), or to spend considerably more on IPV.

Resource-poor countries could not afford the far more expensive IPV, so their choice was to continue with OPV. (As we heard in Chapter 4, it also had other benefits for these nations.) However, resource-rich countries were faced with a dilemma. The argument for persisting with OPV was that the huge extra sum spent on IPV represented an 'opportunity cost'; in other words, they lost the opportunity to spend that money on more effective healthcare intervention – perhaps a different vaccine, or a program to reduce smoking – that would prevent more illness and save more lives. This is a utilitarian argument that says society should make the choice that benefits the most people.

The counter-argument, the one in favour of IPV, says that it is unethical to give a vaccine you know will paralyse children, however few, when a safer vaccine is available. This takes into account the Hippocratic principle of 'First do no harm' (discussed in Chapter 13).

While sitting on the national immunisation committee, I had a protracted albeit respectful disagreement with a public-health colleague about whether Australia should switch from OPV to the far more expensive but safer IPV. Eventually the problem was settled when the price of IPV fell (and that of OPV rose), and IPV was incorporated into a single-injection, six-in-one vaccine with DTP, hepatitis B and Hib.

In reality, the healthcare budget of many countries is not as fixed as is sometimes suggested, and money can be found when a strong case can be made for spending it. Yet healthcare professionals have been nowhere near as successful as, say, the military in persuading governments to spend more on their needs. (I talk more about this issue of vaccine cost in Chapter 14.)

Ensuring vaccine safety

As I consider the tragedies and frauds described in this chapter, I reflect on how little, apparently, they have dented the population's faith in immunisation.

In the early days this was clearly because the diseases were so omnipresent in people's lives. People crippled by polio were everywhere. Parents were prepared to risk the dangers of the early polio vaccines, even after a disaster like the Cutter Incident, because they feared polio even more. In addition, health authorities learned vital lessons from the tragedies, and introduced safeguards that have made it less and less likely that such an error will be made again.

As diseases become rarer, parents who have never seen them depend on their trust of their doctors and nurses. When people become afraid of vaccines and immunisation levels drop, as with whooping cough and measles vaccines in the United Kingdom, the diseases will quickly return and show that parents are correct to trust in vaccines.

In 2011, the WHO introduced a Global Vaccine Safety Initiative to ensure that all countries reach a standard sufficient to ensure vaccine safety. Public health authorities also do surveillance on people receiving long-established vaccines to make sure that if a batch is contaminated, or there has been some unexpected change in the vaccine, it is detected early enough to prevent further damage.

Vaccines have never been safer. Yet as we will discover in the next chapter, that is certainly not everyone's view.

CHAPTER 12

The modern anti-immunisation movement

No rational argument will have a rational effect on a man
who does not want to adopt a rational attitude.

Karl Popper, philosopher (1902–1994)

In his book *Autism's False Prophets*, leading paediatric infection
specialist Paul Offit describes the infamous 2007 Oprah Winfrey
interview with actress Jenny McCarthy on Winfrey's daytime
television show, *Oprah*. When her son Evan was diagnosed with
autism, McCarthy blamed the MMR vaccine. McCarthy said
that Evan was given the vaccine, 'and soon thereafter I noticed
a change. The soul was gone from his eyes.' When Oprah told
her that science suggests MMR vaccine does not cause autism,
McCarthy said: 'My science is Evan, and he's at home. That's my
science.' The audience cheered.

Words have power, and those are powerful words. *Louder Than Words* was the title of McCarthy's book about Evan, and it became a best-seller. At the time McCarthy's partner was the famous actor Jim Carrey, which arguably increased her profile and the amount of attention she received.

McCarthy said her theory was based not on science but 'mommy instinct'. She did her 'research' at the 'University of Google'. According to Offit, the day after the Oprah interview, the national Centers for Disease Control (CDC) was flooded with calls about the safety of MMR vaccine and many paediatricians also fielded inquiries.

Ominous though that sounds, there was no perceptible effect on national uptake of MMR vaccine in the United States. Over 90% of all United States children have been immunised every year since 1996. In 1998, the year Andrew Wakefield's *Lancet* paper was published, there were only 89 cases of measles reported and no deaths.

Wakefield moved to Austin, Texas, in the early 2000s, and has made a living continuing to promote his message that MMR causes autism. His most substantial contribution in his new home State appears to be the network of autism-related charities and businesses with which he has been affiliated, and from some of which he has reportedly drawn six-figure salaries. Wakefield was Executive Director of the Thoughtful House Center for Children in Austin from 2005 to 2010 but resigned after he was struck off the United Kingdom medical register. He founded Strategic Autism Initiative in 2010 with Polly Tommey, a British woman with an autistic son. In 2016, Wakefield directed and Tommey produced a film, *Vaxxed*, which claims there has been a cover-up about vaccine safety at the CDC. Wakefield also founded the

Autism Media Channel in Austin, which produces videos that promote a link between autism and MMR vaccine.

Wakefield credits his popularity in part at least to the rise of social media. Conspiratorial anti-vaccination groups are active on Facebook, and researchers fear this could spread the anti-vaccination movement globally. In the 13 years since Wakefield arrived in Texas, the number of unvaccinated children there has increased almost twenty-fold, from roughly 2300 to 45,000.

Nevertheless, most people in the United States continue to immunise their children with MMR vaccine. Why did the Wakefield scandal have so little effect in the United States? The *Lancet* article, the Deer investigation, the United Kingdom General Medical Council (GMC) inquiry and the other major developments were all local circumstances that resonated more in Britain than overseas. In addition, the American CDC has a strong reputation for expertise regarding infectious diseases and immunisations. The United States also has a strong cohort of paediatric infectious disease experts who were quick to support paediatricians and appear in the mainstream media to debunk myths about MMR vaccine and autism.

Similarly, Australian experts moved swiftly to refute the validity of Wakefield's message in the mainstream media and there was no fall in MMR immunisation rates in Australia. People may be more trusting of their own doctors than of doctors from overseas. A coordinated response by trusted health professionals probably helped undecided parents.

Conflict is integral to human interactions. The mainstream media and social media sometimes talk about immunisation as if opinions are dangerously polarised. If you search the internet for information on the topic, you could be forgiven for thinking opinion is almost equally divided for and against. Is this true? Is polarisation a real problem, or is it exaggerated?

In surveys asking the public which professionals they trust most, nurses usually come top of the list, followed by doctors. Politicians come bottom.

It's just as well that the United States public listens to doctors and nurses rather than politicians on vaccine safety. Donald Trump is notoriously convinced that vaccines cause autism and his willingness to share this belief predates his presidency. His attempts to convey his anti-vaccine message are characteristically inarticulate. In 2014, before he was president, Trump tweeted: 'Healthy young child goes to doctor, gets pumped with massive shot of many vaccines, doesn't feel good and changes – AUTISM. Many such cases!' In 2017, in a conversation with educators, the president said to a teacher in the audience: 'So what's going on with autism? When you look at the tremendous increase, it's really – it's such an incredible – it's really a horrible thing to watch, the tremendous amount of increase.' Trump met Andrew Wakefield in 2016 and the next year Wakefield attended the president's inaugural ball.

Trump's aversion to scientific evidence is illustrated by a 2017 directive to the CDC not to use the terms 'evidence-based' or 'science-based' in reports. Fortunately, the evidence suggests relatively few people in the United States pay attention to Trump's diatribes on vaccines and autism. 'Trust me, I'm a politician' does not seem to have caught on yet, at least as far as vaccine safety is concerned.

Trump's 2014 tweet draws a facile link between the increase in the number of vaccines and the increase in autism. The most likely reason autism has increased so obviously is that we have changed the way we define it.

Leo Kanner, an Austrian-American psychiatrist, wrote the seminal paper first describing autism in 1943. It was called 'Autistic Disturbances of Affective Contact' and described 11 children who were highly intelligent, but displayed 'a powerful desire for aloneness' and 'an obsessive insistence on persistent sameness'. Some of them had 'islands of brilliance', being extraordinarily talented artists or musicians, but they were all very poor communicators, and some were totally mute. With time, the definition of autism expanded to include children who were developmentally delayed.

Recently autism has been reclassified as 'autism spectrum disorder'. As the name suggests, it is now a spectrum that includes children and adults who have difficulties with communication and social interaction, and display restricted or repetitive behaviours and interests. This is a very far cry from Kanner's original narrow definition. In fact, a definition that vague makes me wonder if many of my quirky colleagues don't fulfil those criteria! Probably I do too. As I once wrote, only half in jest, if it's a spectrum, aren't we all on it?

In 2014, the CDC reported a study showing that 1 in 68 United States children (1 in 42 boys and 1 in 189 girls) had been diagnosed with autism spectrum disorder. That means there is one boy with autism in every large United States class.

One extremely unattractive aspect of the recent immunisation controversy has been the fierceness of a very small but vociferous group. In *Autism's False Prophets*, Paul Offit sets out the scientific evidence suggesting MMR vaccine does not cause autism. He has received hate mail and death threats because of his stance. Paul Offit is a courageous man. He does not deserve to be told 'Your day of reckoning is coming' or the even more sinister 'I know where your children go to school.'

It is not clear why autism stimulates such vitriol. If it comes from parents of autistic children, we can at least understand their pain and frustration. If not, there is little excuse.

Why is there scepticism?

Opposition to vaccines is not confined to the autism controversy. In 2008, Jenny McCarthy and Jim Carrey held a rally in Washington DC called 'Green Our Vaccines' to raise awareness of 'toxins' in vaccines. They were photographed wearing green T-shirts bearing that logo. They argued that substances like thiomersal – which we heard about in the previous chapter – cause autism and should be removed from all vaccines. The trouble is that without preservatives, vaccines are more likely to be contaminated and cause infections.

In 2005 Jenny McCarthy founded Generation Rescue, a 'non-profit' organisation that advocates that autism and related disorders are primarily caused by environmental factors, particularly vaccines. Jenny McCarthy certainly seems to have profited from her opposition to vaccines, having published nine books in which she promotes her beliefs.

Considering that medical experts rate immunisation as one of the most important medical advances ever, it is intriguing that there is, and has always been, so much opposition. Part of the reason is rooted in history. When smallpox vaccination was introduced in England in the early 19th century, it was the first major immunisation program in the world. It was a novel idea and public resistance was perhaps unsurprising. As late as 1906, in the preface to his play *The Doctor's Dilemma*, George Bernard Shaw – no lover of the medical profession – called smallpox vaccination 'a particularly filthy piece of witchcraft'.

Nowadays there are anti-vaccination movements in many Western countries, but the extraordinary success of immunisation programs means they lack the widespread appeal of the original anti-vaccination leagues.

Vaccine sceptics and opponents say today – as George Bernard Shaw once did – that putting foreign proteins into our bodies is dangerous and unnatural. They are correct on both counts, but the *extent* to which they are correct requires major qualification.

Firstly, all medicines are potentially harmful and vaccines are no exception. In the last chapter we looked at several occasions in history when vaccines have caused tragic fatalities. While vaccines are getting safer all the time, we should never be blasé about the risks.

Secondly, although the human immune system evolved to cope with foreign micro-organisms and foreign proteins, vaccines include modifications of those organisms that render them immunologically distinct. However, medicine and surgery mainly involve using techniques that could be called 'unnatural'. We use the natural hormone insulin to treat diabetes mellitus, but we modify the insulin (make it 'unnatural') to alter its strength and prolong its effects. If a baby gets stuck during delivery we would perform an 'unnatural' Caesarean section to save the life of both mother and baby. It seems that what is natural and what is unnatural are not very useful concepts in determining what is best for human health.

Julie Leask is an internationally acclaimed social scientist and an associate professor of nursing at the University of Sydney. Professor Leask describes how anti-vaccine parent groups may express antipathy to medical intervention and prefer natural or alternative therapies, such as homeopathy, chiropractic, reflexology and traditional Chinese medicine. They may maintain that a healthy diet is all that is needed to protect their children against infectious diseases. They promote themselves as champions of transparency in public information and of individual choice. They perceive that vaccine companies not only make huge profits from selling vaccines but also exert a pernicious influence on healthcare professionals, research institutes and governments, which for them comprise a 'system' that drives the expansion of immunisation programs.

In general, parents who refuse all vaccines are very unlikely to change their minds. If my colleagues and I look after an unimmunised child in hospital who is critically ill from an infection that would almost certainly have been prevented by routine immunisation, the parents never admit to feeling guilty and almost never agree to let us immunise the child to prevent other infections.

Pru Hobson-West, an English social scientist, describes how a major strategy of vaccine-critical groups is to reframe risk. Doctors preach the need to weigh up the benefits and risks of any medical intervention, including immunisation. The risk of getting life-threatening acute encephalitis from measles is one in a thousand; the risk of getting encephalitis from MMR vaccine is one in a million. To a doctor those figures clearly favour measles immunisation. But a vaccine-critical group will argue that all of us are individuals, which means to them the true risk to each child from vaccines is unpredictable. This emphasis on uncertainty breeds uncertainty. I was recently unable to persuade a father that his child, who had been born without a spleen and was thus at high risk of infection, should be immunised. Although I told him the risk of a life-threatening infection was one in eight and the risk from the vaccine less than 1 in 10,000, he declined to immunise his child, saying he was too worried about vaccine side effects.

Many people, not just committed anti-vaccinationists, fear that giving lots of vaccines might weaken the immune system. They need not worry. The human immune system has evolved to cope with an almost infinite variety of new threats. Indeed, Australian virologist and immunologist Sir Macfarlane Burnet is famous for demonstrating the range and remarkable flexibility of the human immune system.

The most recent evidence suggests that not only do lots of vaccines *not* weaken the immune system, but for some vaccines the complete opposite is true. Professor Julian Higgins and colleagues in Bristol looked at 34 large-scale studies of vaccine impacts and reported their results in the prestigious *British Medical Journal* in 2016. Vaccines against measles and tuberculosis stop children dying from those diseases, but they also stop children from dying from *other* causes over the following two to five years. A child in a developing country who is given a measles-containing vaccine such as MMR vaccine is 25% to 50% less likely to die from *any* cause than a child who does not get measles vaccine. A child in a developing country who is given BCG (anti-tuberculosis) vaccine is 30% less likely to die from *any* cause than a child not given BCG vaccine. We do not know the precise scientific basis for this, but there is little doubt that it is due to stimulation of the child's immune system and of their ability to fight off infections. Of course, it may not be possible to replicate these impressive results in Western countries, where childhood mortality is lower, but they illustrate the point that some vaccines strengthen the immune system and not one has been shown to weaken the immune system.

HPV vaccine scare campaigns

The new human papillomavirus (HPV) vaccine protects against a virus that can cause cervical cancer. HPV vaccine has been the subject of many scare campaigns.

Clinical trials of HPV vaccines in Europe, North America, South America, Asia and Australia published from 2006 onwards found the vaccine was safe and stimulated an immune response, and the vaccine was introduced in Australia in 2007, as we heard in Chapter 7.

In Japan, there was initial enthusiasm, and the uptake of government-funded vaccine by schoolgirls was about 70% in 2013, as it was in Australia. However, media reports of a preliminary (and allegedly fraudulent) mouse study showing the vaccine caused brain damage and unconfirmed video reports of girls in wheelchairs or having convulsions supposedly after receiving the HPV vaccine fuelled anti-vaccine sentiment. Anti-immunisation groups blamed the vaccine for causing chronic body pain and heart and neurological troubles.

Despite a total absence of good evidence of harm, the Japanese Health Ministry hastily suspended the vaccination program pending an investigation. In early 2014, the ministry's panel concluded that there was no evidence the vaccine caused the reported adverse events. However, HPV immunisation rates plummeted from 70% to less than 1% within a year, and the health ministry has never restored its recommendation to give HPV vaccine, even though the vaccine is still government-funded.

Studies worldwide have found that girls report such symptoms just as commonly when unvaccinated as after vaccination with HPV vaccine, and that the vaccine almost never causes serious adverse side effects. European and North American expert reviews agreed the vaccine did not cause the symptoms. The WHO condemned the Japanese Government's risk-averse suspension of their recommendation of HPV vaccine. The WHO's Global Advisory Committee on Vaccine Safety stated pointedly: 'Policy decisions based on weak evidence, leading to lack of use of safe and effective vaccines, can result in real harm.'

Although immunisation levels remain high in Australia, in Denmark and Ireland immunisation levels have fallen, and the adverse publicity from Japan and elsewhere has certainly not helped countries like France, where fewer than 15% of adolescent girls have received the recommended three doses of HPV vaccine. Maybe, as with smallpox vaccine, the eventual success of HPV vaccine will win round the doubters, but it is a tragedy that many young women who will develop cervical cancer could have avoided it through HPV immunisation.

One reason for opposition to HPV vaccine, I believe, is that it relates to an infection that is not classified as a sexually transmitted disease but is nevertheless transmitted through sexual intercourse. United States opposition to HPV vaccine stemming largely from the religious right focused on a strange conviction that girls given the vaccine would be more likely to have sex. One United States mother was quoted as saying, 'I realise it's probably more about my squeamishness with the thought of her becoming sexually active than the vaccination itself. It's not the science. I think it's my own issues around her developing sexually.' Scientific studies show that girls given HPV vaccine are no more likely than girls not given the vaccine to become sexually active, but it is clear that many parents' fear of HPV vaccine really represents their fears around their children's sexual maturity.

British independent broadcaster Joan Shenton, who is also an AIDS denier (someone who does not accept that the HIV virus causes AIDS), made a short anti-HPV vaccine film called *Sacrificial Virgins*. Shenton planned to come to Australia in August 2018 for panel discussions accompanying showings of her film, but had to cancel when the Australian Government did not grant her a visa in time, raising controversy about the balance between freedom of speech and public health. (When our immunisation research workers decided to check out the content, they accidentally found themselves watching an X-rated Nigerian Nollywood film called *The King's Sacrificial Virgins*. The blood-curdling screams of the virgins being sacrificed in gory technicolour echoed around the immunisation department, causing amusement and embarrassment in equal measure.)

After a school-based program was introduced in Australia in 2007, the National HPV Vaccination Program Register recorded that 74% of girls received a full course; the number reached 78% in 2015. After the vaccine was extended to Australian boys, 62% of eligible boys received a full course in 2014 and 70% in 2015. The uptake rate in Australian girls is as high as, and in Australian boys is higher than, anywhere else in the world. In contrast, data from the CDC show that only 18% of eligible teenage girls received a full course when State programs were introduced in the United States in 2008. The numbers rose gradually to 43% for girls and 31.5% for boys in 2016.

Two additional reasons have been put forward for the low uptake of HPV vaccine in the United States compared with Australia. The first involves mainstream and social media.

Katie Couric is an award-winning journalist and author who has worked as a news presenter for three United States television networks. From 2012 to 2014, Couric hosted her own daytime talk show, *Katie*. On 4 December 2013, she hosted an episode entitled 'The HPV Vaccine Controversy'. A promo for the show said: 'The HPV vaccine is considered a life-saving cancer preventer ... but is it a potentially deadly dose for girls? Meet a mom who claims her daughter died after getting the HPV vaccine, and hear all sides of the controversy.'

After the show, Couric was criticised by doctors for airing the anecdotes of people who described adverse events and a death that were probably coincidental and highly unlikely to have been caused by the vaccine. Scientists pointed out that these sorts of stories elicit a strong emotional response in audiences but are a poor way of equipping them to weigh up the risks and benefits of a new vaccine.

A week later Couric apologised – not on air, but in the *Huffington Post* – for giving too much emphasis to adverse events, and pointed out that she had had her own two daughters immunised with HPV vaccine. She wrote:

> The federal government has a system for reporting adverse
> reactions following immunization with any vaccine. For the
> 23 million doses of Gardasil [HPV vaccine] distributed in the
> United States from 2006 to 2008, 12,424 adverse reactions
> were reported, a rate of 5.4 per 10,000 doses, and the vast
> majority of these were minor (transient fever, rash or sore
> arm). Furthermore, only 772 of the 12,424 adverse reactions
> were reported to be serious (persisting symptoms such as
> sore joints, or very rarely a severe allergic reaction called
> anaphylaxis), a rate of 0.3 per 10,000 doses. These rates are
> low compared with other vaccines.

Two weeks after the HPV vaccine show aired, the syndicate announced that *Katie* had been cancelled. They did not say whether it was due to low ratings or the controversy over the vaccine.

It is easy to criticise the mainstream media for poor coverage of immunisation issues (as I have already done in this book). One time a journalist interviewed me over the telephone then asked me for the name of an anti-immunisation advocate. I asked her: if I had been describing the harms of alcohol abuse, would she have asked me for the name of an alcoholic to present the other side of the 'debate'?

To be fair, when Julie Leask performed an in-depth analysis of mainstream news reports in Australia, she found that around 95% were pro-immunisation, which is the same proportion of parents who immunise their children.

People are often concerned that television programs like Katie Couric's have a deleterious effect on HPV vaccine uptake. It is not clear whether or not Jenny McCarthy blaming MMR vaccine for her son's autism on *Oprah* decreased uptake of MMR vaccine or whether Katie Couric's program affected HPV vaccine uptake. But when anti-immunisation views are aired on mainstream media the message is likely to be disseminated on social media.

Does this affect vaccine uptake? Julie Leask and colleagues analysed millions of exposures to Twitter in the United States between 2013 and 2015 and found that media controversies explained 68% of the variance in girls' uptake of the first dose of HPV vaccine. (Other factors known to affect uptake include race, ethnicity, education, income and interactions with the health system.) Tweets about Katie Couric had a particularly high correlation with poor vaccine uptake. Uptake was lower in American States where safety concerns, misinformation and conspiracies comprised a higher proportion of Tweets and correlated better with vaccine uptake than the factors mentioned above. The authors concluded that vaccine coverage is low in States where negative opinions about HPV vaccines are popularised by mainstream media and spread by social media. This does not prove the TV programs *caused* the poor uptake, only that the message spreads and may be used to reinforce anti-vaccination sentiment.

The second reason put forward to explain the difference in uptake of HPV vaccine in Australia and the United States relates to the way the vaccine was introduced in America. The pharmaceutical company Merck applied successfully to the Food and Drug Administration (FDA) to have its HPV vaccine, Gardasil, fast-tracked using a process usually reserved for urgent treatments for serious diseases. This allowed Merck to position itself ahead of its British rival, GSK, which was trying to market its own HPV vaccine, Cervarix. If this fast-tracking had not been approved, Gardasil and Cervarix would have been approved simultaneously by the FDA three years later. Free trade is not necessarily fair trade.

After gaining FDA approval, Merck lobbied State legislatures to add the vaccine to those required for school enrolment. This attempt to politicise the issue of HPV vaccination backfired spectacularly. Political disputes blocked legislative mandates in all but one State. The country became further polarised, dividing according to opinions on whether giving HPV vaccine to girls would encourage them to practise unsafe sex.

No such outcry had accompanied the earlier uneventful introduction of hepatitis B vaccine into United States schools, even though hepatitis B virus can also be transmitted sexually. But hepatitis B vaccine was introduced through the usual public health avenues and family doctors were well informed. In the case of HPV vaccine, Merck's financially driven lobbying bypassed the normal avenues, sidelining public health officials and family doctors in favour of its own marketing.

As we've heard, trust is an essential component of immunisation uptake – particularly when it comes to the introduction of new vaccines. Here trust was taken out of the hands of the family's doctor and invested in an unknown person who told people about the new HPV vaccine in an advertisement. The obvious assumption was that the person in the advertisement was a paid employee of the vaccine company Merck, and that what they said about the vaccine had to be taken in the light of a significant pecuniary conflict of interest.

Misunderstandings about hepatitis B

Since 1982, hepatitis B vaccine has been given to over 500 million people around the world. Its introduction to the United States might not have been controversial, but in France case reports were published suggesting a possible link between hepatitis B vaccine and multiple sclerosis (MS).

MS is a rare condition affecting young adults aged 20 to 40, women more often than men. The cause is unknown, but an abnormal immune response to infection is one theory, although no studies have ever formally connected MS with hepatitis B infection. It is likely the reported link between MS and the vaccine was mere coincidence, due to the large number of hepatitis B vaccine doses given to young adults at the very age when the first symptoms of MS often occur. But that coincidence was difficult to prove.

In 1998, the French Ministry of Health temporarily suspended the school-based adolescent hepatitis B vaccine program while investigations were conducted, but continued to immunise all infants, and adults at special risk.

The French decision was misunderstood and misinterpreted as a ban on all hepatitis B immunisation. Subsequent studies strongly suggest that hepatitis B vaccine does not cause MS. France introduced catch-up immunisation of high school students without mishap. Other countries have routinely continued to immunise adolescents as well as newborns against hepatitis B.

Seeking reliable advice

Trust is a fragile concept in this age when unwelcome facts are dismissed as 'fake news' and scientists are derided. Rumours about harms from immunisation are bound to arise from time to time, and the internet is fertile ground for all sorts of unfounded ideas.

Most people have learned to treat what they read on the internet and social media with suspicion. Why would we put opinion above scientific analysis? On the other hand, if experts disagree, how do we know which ones to trust?

It seems logical to believe the experts we consider the most trustworthy, the most plausible, the most comprehensible and the least likely to be influenced by conflicts of interest. If almost all experts agree, it is improbable that the few dissenting experts are correct.

When asked where they get trustworthy information about immunisation, most people say their family doctor. Trust is one of the key elements in the doctor–patient relationship. Parents generally know and trust their family doctor and rely on him or her to give sound advice. Patients who trust their doctors feel better, behave more healthily and report a better quality of life than those who do not.

There is less polarisation about immunisation than some would have us believe. Most of us *do* trust our doctors, and almost all doctors are pro-immunisation. Most people recognise the benefits of immunisation for their own children and feel good about being part of a community that immunises enough children to prevent the spread of infections. One shot for all, and all for one.

CHAPTER 13

Immunisation and ethics

Recently, when I was on call for cases of paediatric infectious diseases, I was asked to see an infant who was desperately ill with fever, convulsions and shock. The infant had meningitis and survived, but was left with massive brain damage, likely to result in lifelong spastic cerebral palsy.

The mother told one of our young doctors that her child was unimmunised. Meningitis vaccine is included in the routine immunisation schedule, so this child's meningitis and brain damage were almost certainly preventable. The mother's explanation to the stunned young doctor as to why she did not immunise her infant was far from coherent: a friend at church had a baby who'd had a reaction to a vaccine, and some members of the congregation were opposed to immunisation. She was not clear if the church itself was against immunisation, although my inquiries suggest no church group is formally opposed to immunisation.

At this point we were faced with a number of ethical dilemmas. Should we pursue the issue of non-immunisation with the mother? One reason to do so would be to try to persuade her to immunise this infant against infections such as pertussis and influenza that could kill a child with cerebral palsy. A second reason would be to convince her to immunise any future children. A third would be to explore the situation at the church and try to alter the church community's perceptions about immunisation before another disaster occurred.

The danger of discussing it with the mother at that stage was that, whether or not she acknowledged it, she must inevitably feel guilty that her decision had altered the course of her child's life and adversely affected her family's future. That is a huge burden to carry.

Parents in the same situation often appear to deny guilt and say it was fate or God's will. Whether or not the child recovers, they rarely get the child immunised with the vaccines they have missed; presumably to do so would be to admit to having made a bad decision.

It is not a doctor's job to confront people with blame and lay guilt on them; surely that is highly likely to do more harm than good and is, therefore, unethical. Would even raising the subject of immunisation with the mother and listening to what she said be a form of accusation?

There are further ethical considerations. I am writing a book on immunisation and contemplating whether to include this story in a chapter on ethics. Is the story sufficiently identifiable that I would be infringing confidentiality if I did not get the parents' permission before publishing? Is the very way I approached the whole tragic situation with this mother and baby affected by my writing the book? In other words, do I have a significant conflict of interest?

The great Greek physician Hippocrates (whom we've already heard a lot about) deals with confidentiality in the Hippocratic Oath: 'And whatsoever I shall see or hear in the course of my profession, as well as outside my profession in my intercourse with men, if it be what should not be published abroad, I will never divulge, holding such things to be holy secrets.' Health professionals have a moral obligation to respect privacy and confidentiality, and patient confidentiality is something I have considered and endeavoured to preserve whenever I have told clinical stories in this book.

In the end we decided not to discuss immunisation with the mother at the time of her child's acute illness, although for the child's sake we will discuss immunisation with her when she brings her child back for follow-up.

The Hippocratic Oath

Hippocrates is often called the Father of Medicine. He came from the Greek island of Kos and lived roughly 2500 years ago. He founded the Hippocratic School of Medicine, which was instrumental in establishing medicine as a distinct discipline in ancient Greece. Before Hippocrates, medicine and philosophy were intertwined; after Hippocrates, a physician belonged to a separate profession.

As is already evident from the number of distinct diseases he recognised and described, Hippocrates was a brilliant clinician. But even more importantly, Hippocrates and his colleagues developed a code of behaviour for physicians that they enshrined in the Hippocratic Oath. Such depth of thought went into this code that medical students graduating as doctors in most Western countries swear to adhere to modern versions of the same oath. Its principles include:

- agreeing to do the best for one's patients
- avoiding under- and over-treatment
- remembering that there is art to medicine as well as science; warmth, sympathy and understanding may outweigh the surgeon's knife and the chemist's drug
- admitting when one doesn't know
- calling in colleagues for advice when necessary
- respecting patient privacy
- not playing God
- 'preventing disease wherever I can, for prevention is preferable to cure'
- 'remembering that I remain a member of society, with special obligations to all my fellow human beings, those sound of mind and body as well as the infirm'.

These last two – our obligation to prevent disease and to look after everyone in our society – are particularly relevant to immunisation.

Ethics – from the Greek *ethos*, meaning 'habit' or 'custom' – also dates back to the ancient Greek philosophers. Medical philosopher Ian Kerridge has described ethics as the way we feel we ought to behave. This is different from law, which is how we are *permitted* to behave. Ethics affects how all of us conduct our lives, every day. A parent's decision about whether or not to immunise their children has a large ethical component, but so does the way they speak to their children, the way they feed them, the things they allow or don't allow them to do, and so much more.

Doctors and nurses frequently face difficult ethical decisions that may permanently affect their patients and their patients' families. For that reason, medical students and qualified doctors study what health professionals call bioethics – ethics as it relates to health. Studying bioethics does not tell us what to do, but it helps us analyse and reflect on problems in a more structured way than just going with a gut feeling or saying, 'It feels right' or 'It doesn't feel right.'

Hippocrates might have elaborated principles of medical practice 2500 years ago, but some doctors throughout history have decided that those principles did not apply to them. During World War II, the Nazis purged Germany of over 6000 Jewish doctors and used only non-Jewish German doctors. At the end of the war, the United States military held trials of doctors accused of participating in Nazi human experimentation and mass murder. At the first of these, at Nuremberg in 1946, 20 doctors stood trial. Seven were acquitted, four were sentenced to death and hanged, and the rest were sent to prison for 10 to 20 years. Josef Mengele – responsible for some of the worst atrocities, including vicious and often fatal studies on twins – fled from Auschwitz concentration camp to South America and was never captured.

The United States might have accused Nazi doctors of treating Jews as sub-human, but they did not have to look further than their own country for a similar example. From 1932 until 1972, the United States Public Health Service conducted the Tuskegee Study of Untreated Syphilis in the Negro Male. In return for participating in a study of 'bad blood', 431 poor African-American sharecroppers in Alabama known to have syphilis were told they would be given free treatment and free burial insurance (a particularly sinister embellishment). The Public Health Service callously observed, bled and studied the men in order to elucidate the natural history of syphilis. Even after penicillin became available in the 1940s and was known to cure syphilis, the 'Health Service' did not treat either the men or their partners.

The study only came to light through the courage and persistence of a whistle-blower. Peter Buxtun, a Czech-born Jewish social worker and epidemiologist, was 27 when he was employed by the United States Public Health Service in 1965 to interview patients with sexually transmitted diseases. He was appalled when he learned about the Tuskegee experiment. In 1966 Buxtun filed an official protest on ethical grounds.

The Public Health Service ruled that the experiment should continue, because the results were not complete. Buxtun protested again, with the same result. In desperation, he leaked news of the study to the *Washington Post*; the headline news story finally led to the termination of the study in 1972. It was not until 1997 that President Bill Clinton held a ceremony at the White House for survivors of the Tuskegee study, to whom he said:

> What was done cannot be undone. But we can end the
> silence. We can stop turning our heads away. We can
> look you in the eye and finally say on behalf of the
> American people, what the United States government
> did was shameful, and I am sorry ... To our African-
> American citizens, I am sorry that your federal government
> orchestrated a study so clearly racist.

Tainted research

The actions of the Nazis and the doctors at Tuskegee are extreme examples of so-called 'tainted research', in which knowledge is obtained through research that could be seen as unethical.

The different ways in which hepatitis B and hepatitis A are transmitted was elucidated in some highly controversial research undertaken in the 1960s by Dr Saul Krugman and colleagues at Willowbrook. These experiments are famous or infamous, depending on one's view of their ethics, then and now.

Although the name conjures up images of weeping willows and bubbling brooks in verdant pastures, the Willowbrook State School was actually an institution on Staten Island, New York, for children with intellectual disabilities. Saul Krugman and his researchers deliberately infected children with biological material from subjects with hepatitis. The children were either given suspensions of faecal matter to drink or were injected with serum.

While this research had ethics committee approval at the time, and all the children's parents consented to their inclusion in the studies, Dr Krugman and his team were later heavily criticised for being unethical. My scientist father wrote ironically that he had found similar results with his experiments on 'volunteer mice'. Residential places in Willowbrook were scarce and participation in the study gave priority, thus constituting an inducement to enrolment, which ethicists argue constrains choice. However, some doctors argued then and even now that the benefits of the research outweighed the harms to the children.

Most people, when asked whether we should use knowledge from unethical research, think knowledge is knowledge and should not be ignored, although they also say we should make changes to try to prevent unethical research from being conducted in future. Many would condone the use of vaccines originally developed from the research conducted at Willowbrook – but almost no one today would condone the acts perpetrated by the Nazis and at Tuskegee.

Foetal cell lines

There has also been some ethical controversy over the development of several commonly used vaccines because the viruses used to make these vaccines are grown on cell lines derived from embryonic fibroblast cells. Fibroblasts are cells needed to bind skin and connective tissue. Cell lines are kept going for many years by growing them in liquid on the inner surface of glass bottles. After a few days, when the cell layer gets quite thick, the cells are lifted off the surface using a dissolving enzyme such as trypsin, diluted with more liquid and put in extra bottles: a process called 'splitting'.

The original embryonic fibroblast cells used to develop vaccines against hepatitis A, rubella and zoster, and to develop one type of rabies vaccine, came from the elective termination of two pregnancies in the 1960s. The original cell lines, much propagated since, are still in use.

No new foetuses or foetal cells have been involved since the 1960s. But for some people, the original use of foetal tissue means that the vaccine is forever contaminated and should be opposed on ethical grounds.

The Vatican addressed this issue in 2005 in a carefully considered statement, 'Moral Reflections on Vaccines Prepared from Cells Derived from Aborted Foetuses'. It says alternative vaccines should be used if possible, and that pressure should be put on pharmaceutical companies to behave ethically and not put families in morally invidious positions, but that children's health should be the primary concern. It concludes that children and their parents should not be denied vaccines, particularly rubella vaccine, which if not given would result in significant harm to the child, their parents and society.

Hippocrates for the modern era

In the 1970s, in response to atrocities like Tuskegee, the medical profession strove to rediscover the principles of Hippocrates and re-enunciate them in modern terms. After a number of different iterations, United States philosopher Tom Beauchamp and ethicist Jim Childress enunciated in 1977 four commonly used bioethical principles, widely adopted since as guides to how doctors should behave. Of course, being doctors, we give them grandiose names: beneficence, non-maleficence, equity and autonomy.

Beneficence is doing good: a clear moral obligation for all doctors. Non-maleficence is a concept that dates back to the original Hippocratic Oath, and is often expressed using the Latin phrase '*primum non nocere*' (first do no harm). Hippocrates never actually said these words; after all, he spoke Greek, not Latin. But he did say that a physician should promise to 'abstain from doing harm' and promise to 'use treatment to help the sick according to [his or her] ability and judgment, but never with a view to injury and wrong-doing'. Close enough.

Equity is similar to justice; it refers to correcting or attempting to correct a wrong. An equitable distribution of resources implies that money should be spent on competing interests in a fair manner.

Autonomy is often considered the most important principle of all: the right to choose for oneself. The famous 19th century English philosopher John Stuart Mill wrote:

> The only purpose for which power can be rightfully
> exercised over any member of a civilised community, against
> his will, is to prevent harm to others. His own good, either
> physical or moral, is not a sufficient warrant. Over himself,
> over his own body and mind, the individual is sovereign.

A competent individual should be allowed to decide what to do without coercion. This concept is encapsulated in the word 'autonomy' itself: it derives from the Greek for 'self' and 'law'.

Immunisation and autonomy

If we apply Beauchamp and Childress's four principles to immunisation, we can see that it does more good than harm. Like all medical interventions, from taking aspirin to major surgery, vaccines occasionally cause harm, but nowadays they are overwhelmingly safe and effective.

My own view is that people who do not immunise their children are making a poor choice. But the principle of respect for people's autonomy says that we should let them decide for themselves, even if we do not agree with their choices.

There are some interesting points to consider here. Mill expressly specified that we should respect autonomy *as long as it does not do harm to others*. In medicine we take this principle as far as saying that if a mentally competent mother of young children is bleeding to death and we could save her easily with a blood transfusion, but she says no because of a strongly held belief, such as a Jehovah's Witness might hold, we are morally obliged to respect her autonomy. And many of us have had to watch in horror as a young person bled to death when we knew we could save them. Such is the level of respect we hold for the principle of autonomy.

But what about parents' choices when it comes to their children? Society believes that we should usually respect the principle of choice as it applies to the choices parents make about how they raise their children. But children are not their parents' possessions to do with as they like. Children have rights too, and although parents' rights and their children's rights usually coincide, sometimes they differ.

Parents have responsibilities to their children: they are not allowed to harm them to excess, either physically or emotionally. They cannot beat them or sexually assault them or neglect them. If parents make choices that will seriously harm their child, the State reserves the power to intervene. This is the basis of child protection laws.

If a child of Jehovah's Witness parents is in life-saving need of a blood transfusion, doctors will try to persuade the parents first, but if the conflict cannot be resolved the doctors will apply to the courts to over-ride the parents. The courts almost invariably rule for an intervention that will save the child's life, on the grounds that the child is too young to make an autonomous choice, and should be kept alive so they can grow up, in case they would have decided differently to their parents' wishes. John Stuart Mill might have said that the parents' decision *does* harm another, namely their child, and so their right to make the decision about the child's transfusion is forfeit.

Does the assertion that Jehovah's Witness children need to be able to grow up to make their own decisions also apply to immunisation? In some countries this is one of the reasons given for compulsory immunisation: a child who is damaged by or even dies from a preventable infection might have chosen to be immunised if allowed to grow up and make their own choice.

However, the counter-argument is that we generally trust parents to make good choices regarding their children's healthcare. This is not because parents own their children, but because most parents love their children, will try to make wise choices on their behalf and will have to live with the consequences if those choices turn out badly.

Doctors and other members of society are very reluctant to interfere with parental decision-making about their children's health. For this reason, in many places, including Australia, the United Kingdom and many American States, routine childhood immunisation is optional, not compulsory. But there are specific situations regarding immunisation in which the risks to the child from not immunising are *greater*, and the usual rules about parental choice and compulsion may not apply.

In 2009, I was consulted about a newly born baby whose mother was known to have chronic hepatitis B infection; she and the baby's father had refused to allow doctors to immunise the baby. Historically, between a quarter and a third of all people with chronic hepatitis B infection have died young because they developed cirrhosis of the liver or liver cancer. The prognosis is better with modern medicine, but chronic hepatitis B is still a serious infection with lifelong implications. The risk that a baby will develop chronic hepatitis B infection from its mother varies according to how active the mother's infection is.

In this case, the mother's infection was relatively quiescent and the risk to the baby without any intervention was 10% (a 1 in 10 chance). However, we knew that injecting the baby with hepatitis B vaccine (and giving an injection of antibody at birth to mop up any virus and increase the protection) would reduce the risk to 1% (a 1 in 100 chance). There is ample evidence that both the vaccine and the immunoglobulin (antibody) are extremely safe. We tried to persuade the parents to let us protect their baby, but they were adamant in their belief that the aluminium in the vaccine was toxic and would be harmful. We pointed out that if their child caught hepatitis B, they would be at greatly increased risk of liver cancer, a risk which could probably have been prevented by the vaccine. The parents did not change their minds.

Although routine childhood immunisation is not mandatory in Australia, in this particular, non-routine situation the risk was much higher than normal. We explained that we would be prepared to ask a judge for a court order to make their baby a ward of court. The parents would be allowed to make their case for no immunisation to the court and the court would decide on the merits of the case. If we were successful, the baby would remain with the parents but the court would rule that health authorities could immunise the baby.

The parents still did not agree to immunisation. We decided we had a duty to try to protect the infant. Because the proposed intervention was very safe and minimally invasive, and the outcome if the baby became infected was serious and could quite possibly shorten the baby's life significantly, we felt justified in asking a court to decide whether or not it was reasonable to over-rule the parents to protect their child.

We went to court and won the case, but it was a pyrrhic victory. The parents left the hospital secretly and went on the run with the baby and a three-year-old sibling, evading child protection staff and making frequent phone calls to the media saying, 'The doctors are infringing our rights.' Anti-immunisation lobby groups championed their cause. We pointed out that the baby had rights too, and that in this case the parents' and the baby's rights were in conflict, and that *the court* had ruled that the baby's rights took precedence, not us.

The vaccine and immunoglobulin are usually given at birth, ideally within two to three days of birth; the greater the delay the less effective they will be because the virus will have infected the baby. After the family had been on the run for a week, it was probably too late to immunise the child, and the authorities quietly dropped the pursuit.

Although the baby in this case was never given hepatitis B vaccine, there were some positive aspects of the case. It set a legal precedent, so that when similar cases have gone to the Australian courts since, the court has usually ruled in favour of the doctors. (In contrast, in an identical situation, a New Zealand court ruled in favour of the parents.)

On the few subsequent occasions when my colleagues and I have faced similar situations, we have been able to tell the parents that we are prepared to go to court, and that precedent suggested we would probably win. Confronted with this knowledge, the parents I have counselled have all decided to have their children immunised against hepatitis B. I have been able to continue seeing the baby and the parents in clinic in an atmosphere of mutual respect, giving the baby each dose of hepatitis B vaccine while respecting the parents' decision about other routine childhood vaccines.

There are special situations in which the risk of non-immunisation is even higher than with maternal hepatitis B. For example, a child who catches rabies after being bitten or scratched by a rabid animal (for example, a raccoon in the United States, a dog or a monkey in Asia, or a bat in Australia) is virtually certain to die, unless they are given vaccine soon after the injury. If the parents refused the vaccine, almost everyone would see it as a child protection issue and the courts would rule that the child must be made a ward of court and given the vaccine.

The diseases prevented by routine childhood immunisation are now sufficiently rare that the risk that a normal unimmunised child will develop one of them and be severely harmed is in fact very low. This is why we as a society feel able to let parents decide whether or not their children should receive routine childhood immunisations.

Immunisation and other people's rights

Of course, a decision not to immunise has an impact beyond the individual child and their parents. Other parents may well say: 'If you do not immunise *your* child, you are being selfish and putting *my* child at risk. You talk about *your* right to decide, but what about *my* child's right to be healthy?'

If all the children but one or two in a child care facility or school are immunised, the unimmunised children will be protected through herd immunity. But if lots of parents decide not to immunise their children, infections will spread through the population. This was starkly illustrated by outbreaks of measles in Europe in 2017, resulting in at least 35 deaths – 31 in Romania, two in Italy and one each in Germany and Portugal.

Measles vaccine is 95 to 98% effective, so when measles is circulating, up to 1 in every 20 immunised children will still catch it. Their parents will be understandably critical of the 'selfish' parents who permit measles to circulate. They may see them as 'freeloaders' who allow their children to be protected by other immunised children without incurring any risk or effort.

We are all members of communities, and as such we have some obligations to others, although opinions will vary as to the extent of these obligations. Do we have a moral obligation to get our children immunised to protect other children at their child care facility or school?

The measles outbreaks in some European countries have been blamed on falling uptakes of childhood measles vaccine following the MMR–autism scare described in Chapter 11. Italy, where there were more than 3000 cases of measles in 2017, thereafter banned unimmunised children from attending State schools, with fines and even removal of the child from parental custody as penalties for non-compliance. In Romania, where an outbreak of measles infected over 6000 people in less than a year and killed 31 children, draft legislation making immunisation against measles compulsory was hotly debated due to public opposition. In the United Kingdom, however, where the autism saga originated, measles immunisation levels recovered without legislation.

Making immunisation compulsory has two big problems. As well as infringing parents' freedom to make their own health choices, it may alienate people who feel they are not trusted to choose wisely. Arguably, people are more likely to value immunisation and to trust the medical profession regarding vaccine safety if they are allowed to choose whether or not to immunise their children. Compulsion – as with smallpox vaccine in the 19th century in the United Kingdom and the United States – may well generate opposition. It also engenders suspicion. If a vaccine is safe and effective, why do we need to make it compulsory?

If immunisation *is* made compulsory, there will need to be sanctions for parents who refuse it, and these sanctions should surely be proportionate. In Belgium in 2008, two sets of parents were fined and sentenced to imprisonment for five months for refusing to allow their children to undergo compulsory polio immunisation. In practice, the sentence was suspended and the parents decided that polio vaccine was preferable to prison. Such a punitive approach literally threatens to infringe the parents' liberty, and is almost certain to entrench anti-immunisers in their beliefs about the iniquity of State intervention.

The risk of contracting a particular infection, the risk of serious harm for children who *do* contract the infection and the risk from the vaccine will vary from infection to infection. The risk that Belgian children would catch or transmit polio in 2008 was negligible, so the Belgian Government's decision to introduce legislation making polio immunisation – but not other immunisations – compulsory was puzzling. Their decision to threaten parents who dissented with imprisonment was even more contentious. Perhaps they were trying to make a point, but the rationale was questionable and the implementation heavy-handed, and there is a danger that such incidents will stimulate more outraged opposition than could be justified by any slight temporary improvement in immunisation rates.

Many jurisdictions have passed laws allowing child care facilities and schools to exclude unimmunised children during an outbreak of measles or whooping cough in order to protect other immunised children; this seems a good compromise. In Australia, many States have gone further, and introduced a policy banning any unimmunised children from attending child care centres and after-school care, colloquially called 'No Jab No Play'.

Australia's national 'No Jab No Pay' legislation also requires children to be fully immunised for parents to be eligible for the Family Tax Benefit, Child Care Benefit and Child Care Rebate. This could be seen as an incentive by those who approve of immunisation, or as a punishment by those who disapprove: carrot or stick. The big risk is that the legislation penalises socially disadvantaged parents who do not get their children immunised because of circumstances, not ideology.

Most parents in Australia immunise their children as a result of education, not compulsion, so resorting to legislation could be seen as unnecessary and disrespectful of people's freedom to choose. The counter-argument is that legislation is effective in improving immunisation rates, and that as long as there is exemption for conscientious objectors, 'No Jab No Pay' and 'No Jab No Play' are ethically justifiable. Australian law makes parents put seat-belts on their children in cars. An injection is a bit more invasive and the risks from an immunisation are a bit higher, but the ethical difference constituted by these matters of degree is debatable.

In 2017, a well-nourished, healthy seven-year-old girl cut her foot while playing in the garden. In her northern New South Wales town, only 70% of children are immunised by age five, compared with over 93% nationally. Like 30% of children in her 'alternative' community, she was unimmunised.

Her parents cleaned her foot thoroughly, but within days she developed excruciating spasms in her leg, followed by spasms in other muscles and had difficulty breathing, all caused by tetanus. She was treated for some weeks in a paediatric intensive care unit, with a tube inserted down her trachea to give artificial ventilation to save her life.

Vaccine advocates called the girl's parents irresponsible; anti-vaccination groups blamed the doctors for not diagnosing the girl's symptoms more quickly. Australia reports two to seven cases of tetanus a year, but only in unimmunised children and elderly adults.

The parents' decision not to immunise this poor girl cost her a great deal of pain, an intensive care admission and, nearly, her life. In addition, her intensive care stay cost the government, and thus taxpayers, a great deal of money. Occasional disasters like this raise questions about compulsory immunisation or suggestions that the parents should be charged for the hospital stay. But if we believe in a public health service and in respecting parental choice in general, we should have second thoughts about such punitive measures.

'Altruistic immunisation'

Some vaccines are given not primarily to protect the child but to protect others. One example is rubella vaccine for boys. As we've heard, Australia now immunises boys as well as girls against rubella, not to protect the boys, who would only ever catch a mild infection, but to stop the virus from circulating and to protect women of child-bearing age. This means that boys also benefit, because they are less likely to have daughters or sons or nieces or nephews with the horrible condition of congenital rubella syndrome. The parents of young boys already accept the tiny risk of harm in order to protect society from rubella. Any society would want to help families avoid having a baby with this condition.

A second example of 'altruistic immunisation' is giving human papillomavirus (HPV) vaccine to boys. The vaccine protects them against penile warts, and may protect them against anal cancer, which affects mainly men who have sex with men, and against penile cancer, which is exceedingly rare. HPV vaccines may also protect against some oropharyngeal cancers (cancers of the throat tissues), although this remains contentious and unproven. But the main rationale is to help protect girls against cervical cancer.

As with rubella vaccine, boys and society derive benefit if women avoid cervical cancer, but a degree of altruism is involved in immunising boys against an infection for a mostly secondary benefit. There is a difference with the rubella situation, in that we give MMR vaccine at one to four years of age when children's consent is not sought, whereas we usually give HPV vaccine to 12- or 13-year-old boys, who might reasonably be involved in the consent process. The high uptake among Australian boys suggests they are willing to receive an injection to protect girls, so maybe altruism is alive and kicking.

What about immunisation for healthcare workers? It seems reasonable to expect them to be vaccinated in order to protect their patients from catching an infection. Most healthcare workers agree, but the evidence that it actually protects patients is poor – even in the case of cancer patients with greatly weakened immune systems. However, there is certainly an argument for making it a condition of employment that staff working with immunocompromised patients be immunised against the most transmissible organisms – influenza, hepatitis B, whooping cough, measles and chickenpox – at the very least. Unimmunised staff could be compulsorily redeployed to other areas.

In 2013, an Indiana hospital sacked eight employees, including three experienced nurses, for refusing influenza immunisation, which the hospital had made mandatory for all employees. Ethel Hoover, aged 61, wore all black on her last day of work as an intensive care nurse, saying she was in mourning because she had been at the hospital almost 22 years and had only been off sick four or five days in her whole career. 'This is my body. I have a right to refuse the flu vaccine,' she said. Her hospital had sacked her rather than let her move to a less critical area, which might have been a fair compromise.

Is the patient's right to be protected more important than the healthcare worker's autonomy? The argument against mandatory immunisation of healthcare workers, much like the argument against compulsory routine childhood immunisations, is that it is preferable to persuade than to punish. Compulsion would hold more weight if there were stronger evidence that immunising staff actually protects patients, but the reality is that most patients get infected by family and friends, not staff.

One of the main reasons some healthcare workers do not get their annual influenza immunisation is lack of opportunity. We are all short of time, and we all hate paying for things. If vaccines are free and easily available in the workplace, most staff get themselves immunised.

Immunisation and compensation

Societies that expect parents to immunise their child to protect that child and to protect other members of society arguably have a moral obligation to provide compensation in the rare event that the child suffers a serious adverse effect. Suppose a child who received OPV were to be the unlucky 1 out of 2.5 million children given OPV who is paralysed by the vaccine? What do we owe the child and family?

If the country has an efficient public health service, it could be argued that the paralysed child will be cared for by the free health system. Yet the health system cannot compensate for the emotional cost to the child and the family or the lost life opportunities, let alone all the additional financial expenses incurred.

In 1986, the United States Congress decided on an innovative solution to protect vaccine manufacturers against litigation: they introduced a National Vaccine Injury Compensation Program. It was an attempt to deal with the worrying trend of increasing numbers of opportunistic lawsuits against vaccine manufacturers, which they feared would impair the development of new vaccines. Under this program, manufacturers of vaccines pay a tax to the United States Treasury of 75 cents on each dose of vaccine. If someone thinks a vaccine covered by the program (which includes all routine childhood immunisations and some adult ones) has damaged them or their child, they cannot sue a vaccine manufacturer without first filing a claim with the United States Court of Federal Claims. A determination is made by the court as to whether or not the claim is valid. The claimant can only sue the vaccine company if the claim is rejected or if the claimant rejects any compensation offered.

In 1961, Germany introduced a no-fault compensation scheme for injuries thought likely to be related to immunisation. By 2005, 18 other countries had introduced similar schemes. The benefits provided include medical costs, disability pensions and compensation for emotional harms. Most of the schemes are conducted under the aegis of State or national governments, except in Finland and Sweden, where they are coordinated by pharmaceutical manufacturers. Decisions on which possible vaccine-related injuries should be compensated are made using pre-established criteria or are assessed on a case-by-case basis, but the standard of proof is usually lower than for court cases.

Australia has no such vaccine injury compensation scheme, although many public health advocates and ethicists believe it should. I am one of those who has tried unsuccessfully for years to persuade the Australian Government to set up a compensation scheme as the ethical thing to do. The government has put it in the too-hard basket. They now say the new National Disability Insurance Scheme (NDIS) will provide support for anyone with likely vaccine-related injury, but we are yet to see if the support will be adequate.

Social trust

Having trusted sources of information – usually the family doctor – helps parents make informed decisions about whether immunisation is safe for their children. However, there is an important interplay between this interpersonal trust and the concept of social trust. The latter refers to trust in collective institutions, including the government and public health bodies, and is influenced by the mainstream and social media.

Governments and health professionals need to earn that trust and maintain it by ensuring that vaccines and immunisation programs are as safe and effective as possible. This places an obligation on them to monitor the safety of new vaccines, and to be open and honest with the public about any problems that emerge.

There is overwhelming evidence that immunisation is a potent cause of falling levels of infectious diseases, and that vaccines have never been safer. If the public remains assured of these things, social trust will be maintained and immunisation levels will remain high. High immunisation levels obtained through trust will obviate the need for harsh interventions to ensure children are immunised. This in turn will mean parents feel the government trusts their ability to make wise decisions for their children.

CHAPTER 14

Overcoming the iniquity of poverty

In 2017, a boy in East Timor with advanced cancer presented to a paediatrician working for a charity. In the paediatrician's homeland, the boy would have received the latest chemotherapy medicines and had a modest chance of survival. But these medicines were not available in East Timor. The paediatrician persuaded the East Timorese Ministry of Health to fund the chemotherapy. A public health physician commented bitterly, 'There goes my whole immunisation budget for the year.'

A person born in a Western country today can expect to live 25 years longer than someone born in the same country a century ago. This remarkable change in life expectancy is due to multiple factors, including antibiotics and clean water, but immunisation has certainly contributed significantly. The WHO estimates that 2 to 3 million lives are saved each year due to immunisations.

However, the WHO also estimates that 1.5 million children under five years old still die each year due to a vaccine-preventable disease; almost all of them live, and die, in developing countries. Parents in first-world countries agonise about the safety of childhood vaccines at the same time as parents in third-world countries are mourning the loss of their child from a vaccine-preventable infection.

There are two major barriers to immunising children in poor countries. The first is the inability to make better use of existing vaccines, which are not being given because of lack of money or health infrastructure. The second is the lack of availability of vaccines against infections like malaria or dengue fever, which occur almost exclusively in developing countries. This lack of availability is due at least partly to the fact that vaccine companies hesitate to develop vaccines that will not generate profits for them.

Expanding immunisation to the world

Donald Ainslie (DA) Henderson led the WHO's global Intenstive Smallpox Eradication Programme from 1967 and eliminated smallpox from the world within a decade (see Chapter 2). When asked what should be eradicated next, DA usually said, 'Bad management.' That caustic comment belied the fact that his contribution to immunisation extended way beyond smallpox.

While his team was delivering smallpox vaccine in parts of Africa and Asia, DA was struck by the fact that almost no children in those places were receiving the childhood vaccines routinely given to children in his native America and in other Western countries. Surely, he reasoned, something could and should be done about this. In the *Bulletin of the World Health Organization* he is quoted as saying: 'We found very quickly that in Africa the average vaccinator could reach 500 African children a day. We wondered "Why aren't we doing this with more vaccines?"' It took seven years from 1967 for DA to convince others in the WHO to act.

In 1974, as I was nearing the end of my medical training and soon to become a real doctor, I did a two-month student elective in a mission hospital in the small town of Moshi in Tanzania, at the foot of Mount Kilimanjaro. There I saw wards of children dying from the complications of measles despite the antibiotics we gave them. Some of them were malnourished, but most of them were a good weight and had previously been healthy. That year, fewer than 5% of children in developing countries received a third dose of DTP and poliomyelitis vaccines in their first year of life, and almost no child received measles vaccine. That year, over a million children died from measles in Africa alone. That year, the widespread use of measles vaccine in the United States, which had started in 1968 and was ramped up in 1973, ensured that only 20 children died from measles throughout the entire country. So much for global equity.

It was also in 1974 that the WHO finally heeded DA Henderson's urging and established its Expanded Programme on Immunization (EPI). The EPI's aim was to radically improve the global uptake of vaccines against six major diseases: diphtheria, tetanus and pertussis (DTP vaccine), polio, measles and tuberculosis.

This was a laudable aim, but there was a major problem: the program was seriously under-funded. The EPI's first full-time director, Dr Ralph (Rafe) Henderson – not related to DA – later said it 'sputtered along with only one full-time medical officer and secretary, supplemented by part-timers lent from other divisions'. Worse, it did not come with any funding for developing countries, so each country had to pay for its own vaccines, and for the healthcare systems needed to deliver the vaccines to children. Progress was difficult due to enormous logistical problems, including extreme poverty, poor health infrastructure, remote populations, poor roads and transport, and failure of the 'cold chain' (vaccines can be destroyed if they overheat). War and famine in many countries in Africa and Asia further compromised the already difficult task.

Dr Halfdan Mahler (1923–2016) was a Danish physician, and WHO Director-General on three separate occasions between 1973 and 1988, and also a pioneer of social justice. In 1977, when the EPI was stagnating, Mahler committed over a million dollars of the WHO's regular budget to allow the program to employ eight professional and four secretarial staff. He is widely acclaimed for being instrumental in organising the Declaration of Alma-Ata, signed by the WHO, the United Nations Children's Fund (UNICEF) and 134 nations in 1978. It was one of the most significant moments in public health history. Under the banner 'Health for All by 2000', the declaration established health as a fundamental human right. On the 30th anniversary of the Declaration of Alma-Ata in 2008, Mahler said: 'Unless we all become partisans in renewed local and global battles for social and economic equity in the spirit of distributive justice, we shall indeed betray the future of our children and grandchildren.'

In the mid-1970s few developing countries had immunisation programs. Most just responded to outbreaks as they occurred. Ciro de Quadros, who had been so courageous in the elimination of polio from Ethiopia in 1971 (see Chapter 4), was appointed head of EPI in the Americas in 1976. His first step was to persuade individual countries to appoint a national immunisation manager. De Quadros later explained:

> We brought together the country managers and everyone
> else from the governments working in epidemiology, primary
> health care, and so on, and listed the problems – how to
> improve coverage, do surveillance and organise the cold
> chain – and analysed them. Then we worked on each
> problem and solution in each country.

But the big leap forward in immunising the poor children of the world came when the United Nations Children's Fund became heavily involved.

The role of UNICEF

UNICEF had been established by the United Nations after World War II to help children facing famine and infections in war-devastated countries. From 1950, UNICEF broadened its focus to include all developing countries. UNICEF relied heavily on aid contributions from industrialised countries, which provided two-thirds of all its funds. The rest came from private donors.

In 1954, the movie star Danny Kaye became UNICEF's Goodwill Ambassador. It was an inspired choice. Danny Kaye was the first celebrity in the world to advocate for a global cause. Instantly recognisable at the time for his gangling dancing, his high-pitched voice and his carefully crafted slapstick comedy, Kaye loved to be with children and was loved by them in turn. He travelled the world for UNICEF, raising awareness and funds, and made a promotional film called *Assignment Children* about UNICEF's work in Asia, which was watched by over 100 million people. Describing his work with UNICEF, he later said: 'I believe deeply that children are more powerful than oil, more beautiful than rivers, more precious than any other natural resource a country can have. I feel that the most rewarding thing I have ever done in my life is to be associated with UNICEF.'

UNICEF also played an integral role in developing the Declaration of the Rights of the Child, which was adopted by the United Nations in 1959. For this and other work, UNICEF won the 1965 Nobel Peace Prize for 'the promotion of brotherhood among nations'.

It was not until 1980, when James P Grant (1922–1995) was appointed as executive director, that UNICEF's involvement in worldwide vaccination took off. A visionary and a passionate proponent of low-cost, practical solutions, Grant immediately set about making himself one of the most important figures ever in global child health. He gave direction and urgency to UNICEF.

Grant called the parlous state of the health of the world's children a 'global silent emergency'. He focused on three major issues. The first was gastroenteritis, which at the time killed more than 5 million children a year. The solution was just that: oral rehydration solution (ORS), made from adding water to the right quantities of sugar and salt. The second issue was breastfeeding: the WHO and UNICEF's Baby-Friendly Hospital Initiative was launched in 1991. And the third major focus was immunisation. UNICEF made a major contribution to the EPI by providing specially designed refrigerators and cold boxes to maintain the cold chain. They also provided syringes, needles and sterilisers to aid vaccine delivery.

Grant believed it was important to measure the successes and sometimes the failures of the initiatives instituted by UNICEF. He initiated a report, first released in 1996, called 'The State of the World's Children', which is still published annually. It documents information not only on immunisation, but also on other diverse topics relating to childhood. Just before Grant died from cancer aged 72, President Bill Clinton sent him a letter that thanked him 'from the bottom of my heart for your service to America, to UNICEF and most of all to the children of the world'.

Under Grant, the WHO set itself an ambitious target of immunising all the world's children by 1990. Although this goal was unrealistic, it was aspirational. In practice, UNICEF reported that in 1990, 76% of the children in the world received three doses of DTP vaccine and 73% of children received measles vaccine, compared with fewer than 5% of them receiving a full course of DTP or measles vaccine just 16 years earlier in 1974.

This was a remarkable achievement. However, progress for the next few years after 1990 was slow. The numbers stopped rising at anything like the previous rate, and public health experts began to talk of 'vaccine fatigue'. I visited Uganda to teach paediatric infectious diseases to young doctors on three occasions between 1990 and 1997, and on each occasion, despite the efforts to introduce immunisation, I saw newborn babies with their faces and limbs rigid with tetanus, and young children dying from severe measles. Health clinics were operating, but HIV infection had hit Uganda and I saw many mothers, infants and older children with AIDS.

When HIV began to spread, health services in many developing countries had to commit scarce resources to trying to treat and prevent infection, and immunisation services took a lower priority. Parents with AIDS are often too ill to get their children immunised, and children with AIDS do not respond as well to vaccines.

It was not until Bill and Melinda Gates started GAVI, the Global Alliance for Vaccines and Immunization, that global immunisation got back on track. That was the year 2000, and it heralded the start of a hopeful new millennium.

Philanthropy and immunisation

Having children made us look differently at all these things
that we take for granted, like taking your child to get a
vaccine against measles or polio.

Melinda Gates, philanthropist (born 1964)

Americans have a long record – of which they are justifiably proud – of improving access to vaccines through philanthropy. One early example was the March of Dimes (discussed in Chapter 4), the not-for-profit organisation started in 1938 by President Franklin D Roosevelt (FDR) to combat polio. Polio vaccines were not developed with resource-poor countries in mind, but there is no doubt that the March of Dimes has contributed significantly to the global near-eradication of polio.

While the March of Dimes subsequently shifted its emphasis to birth defects and to improving infant mortality, the organisation funded a rubella immunisation program in the 1970s to prevent congenital rubella syndrome, and as recently as 2010 promoted adult pertussis immunisation to protect infants against whooping cough. The primary focus of the March of Dimes has been to improve the health of all people in the United States, rich and poor alike, but the benefits for children in poor countries have been enormous.

The charity Rotary has also played a major role in improving immunisation rates, initially for polio vaccine, but subsequently for other vaccines as well. The first ever Rotary Club meeting was held in downtown Chicago in 1905, when a lawyer, Paul Harris, met with three business acquaintances, a coal merchant, a tailor and an engineer. Their aim was to create a network of businessmen to foster ethical behaviour and good works. They kept on meeting regularly, and called themselves Rotary because they rotated the meetings from one person's office to another.

Rotary Clubs sprang up in the United States and beyond. In 1922, the organisation became known as Rotary International. By 1925 there were 200 clubs and over 20,000 members.

Clem (later Sir Clem) Renouf was born in the small North Queensland sugar-cane town of Ingham and became an accountant. He was keen to contribute to society beyond the sugar plantations of Queensland. In 1950 a Rotary Club was started in the neighbouring town of Nambour and a friend invited Renouf along. He joined and eventually rose through the ranks to be elected President of Rotary International in 1978.

As his year-long term neared its end, Renouf heard the wonderful news of the global eradication of smallpox, and wondered if Rotary could lead the next great eradication campaign. He rang Dr John Sever, Head of Infectious Diseases at the prestigious National Institutes of Health in Washington DC and a Rotary district officer. Sever rang back two days later to say that polio was maiming over a thousand children a day in the world. Eradicating polio should be Rotary's target.

In 1979 Rotary went into partnership with the Philippines to improve their rates of polio immunisation. In 1985 Rotary launched PolioPlus, a global program with the aim of eradicating polio. The program was possible because workers with almost no training could drip oral polio vaccine into children's mouths. From 1995, Rotary and the Indian Government joined in a prototype partnership between an altruistic charity and a national government to achieve the almost unthinkable: India is now free of polio.

Rotary didn't rest on its laurels in India. The WHO's EPI had recommended that all children in developing countries receive vaccines against seven diseases – diphtheria, tetanus, pertussis, polio, tuberculosis, measles and hepatitis B – but India was struggling to achieve this. In 2009, only 61% of Indian children were immunised against all seven diseases, and only 65% in 2013.

In 2014, on Christmas Day, also known as Good Governance Day in India, the Indian Health Minister launched Mission Indradhanush. Indradhanush means rainbow in Hindi, and the seven colours of the rainbow represent seven diseases – the six EPI infections plus hepatitis B. Rotary and the Indian Government are again collaborating to try to get these EPI vaccines to India's poorest children, and have set an ambitious target of 100% coverage by the year 2020. If they can get anywhere near that, they will have saved many thousands of lives.

Another contemporary example of United States philanthropy directed specifically at poor countries is the Bill and Melinda Gates Foundation. Bill Gates co-founded Microsoft in 1975 and made a massive fortune from the computer industry, becoming one of the richest men in the world. There have been many billionaires in the world who have done great good with their fortunes. John and Laura Rockefeller's foundation promotes education. Solomon and Peggy Guggenheim's foundation promotes the arts. But I cannot think of anyone besides Bill Gates who has so successfully devoted his money, mind and soul to combating the effects of poverty in developing countries.

Many credit Melinda Gates with being the driving force behind the charitable distribution of Gates's fortune and the establishment and administration of the foundation. Yet researchers close to the couple say Bill is equally committed to using his fortune to save as many lives as possible. However the credit is attributed, the Gateses make an extraordinary couple and both deserve the highest praise for their efforts to overcome global health inequity.

The Bill and Melinda Gates Foundation was launched with millennial fervour in January 2000, and in the 15 years to the end of 2014 contributed US$44.3 billion to improving the health of children in developing countries. Bill and Melinda are brilliant at seeking and taking advice on the best way to direct their funds in order to have the maximum impact on improving the health of people in poor countries.

Inspired by the Gateses' example, another United States billionaire, businessman Warren Buffett, has given away 99% of his fortune, most of it to the Bill and Melinda Gates Foundation.

One of the major aims of the foundation has been to improve global immunisation rates, and to this end, also in January 2000, it launched GAVI, the Global Alliance for Vaccines and Immunization (now just called Gavi, the Vaccine Alliance). Gavi is an innovative partnership between the public and private sectors, designed to reduce inequities in vaccine delivery and development.

It aims at sustainability by co-funding immunisation programs and using the demonstrated benefits to convince governments to continue funding the programs when Gavi withdraws.

Gavi also negotiates competitive prices with vaccine companies by offering to buy vaccines in enormous quantities if the companies reduce their price. For example, in 2013 Gavi was able to make HPV vaccine, which costs over US$100 a dose in some industrialised countries, available for US$4.50 a dose in developing countries that could afford that price. By the end of 2016, HPV vaccine had been introduced in 74 countries.

This is a win-win situation. The vaccine company does not lose money even though the price is much lower, while the people in developing countries also benefit. If the vaccine company can sell the same vaccine at a far higher price to industrialised countries and make a sizeable profit, which allows it to be 'altruistic', then industrialised countries can feel that they too have played a role in making the vaccine available to the poor.

Hepatitis B vaccine cost more than US$70 a dose when first manufactured in the 1980s, and still costs around $25 a dose in industrialised countries, even more in the private sector. But it is sometimes sold wholesale for less than $1 a dose (sometimes as low as 58 cents a dose) to developing countries in Asia with a very high incidence of hepatitis B infection. By the end of 2016, 186 countries had introduced routine hepatitis B vaccine for infants. The WHO estimates that 84% of infants in the world received three doses of hepatitis B vaccine in 2016, and as many as 92% in the Western Pacific.

Gavi has also made a major contribution to improving measles vaccine availability in developing countries, and estimates that 5.5 billion doses have been given since the year 2000. It is truly ironic that in 2016, as European countries struggled with falling measles immunisation rates due to vaccine controversies, the WHO announced that the global number of measles deaths had fallen below 100,000 in a year for the first time in history. This compares with 2.6 million deaths a year in the 1980s. It is a perfect illustration of how some industrialised countries have become fixated with viewing vaccines from a political perspective, while developing countries can see that those same vaccines will save their children's lives.

By 2015, Gavi had immunised 500 million children, and 7 million deaths had been prevented. It aims to immunise an additional 300 million children by 2020, which will prevent a further 5 to 6 million deaths. The WHO's latest target of 90% coverage with all recommended childhood vaccines by 2020 – much more realistic than its original target of 100% coverage by 1990 – is achievable.

What a remarkable legacy for the estimable Bill and Melinda Gates (and those like Warren Buffett who have been inspired by their example). Few if any rich people will ever make better use of their fortunes.

Foreign aid

A cynical view says that wealthy countries give foreign aid to poor countries to gain an economic and political foothold in places that are rich in natural resources and of strategic significance. But when David Cameron became British Prime Minister in 2010, his government took a strong stand against that attitude. Andrew Mitchell, his International Development Secretary, famously declared: 'We will not balance the books on the backs of the world's poorest people. Britain will keep its promise to them.' Even as Cameron's Conservative government was making cuts to domestic spending, he said they would 'ringfence' the foreign aid budget.

Shoring up his position on this in *The Observer* on 12 June 2011, David Cameron wrote:

Tabitha Mukhali is 32 years old. She lives in Kibera, a slum in Nairobi, Kenya. Last year her eldest son, John, contracted pneumonia. For a month he lay in agony, battling the disease; no one could help him. It was a fight ultimately that he did not win. He was just a year old. But now there's new hope for mothers like Tabitha. In January this year a new pneumococcal vaccine was introduced to Kenya.

Cameron went on to describe how some of the cost of the vaccine and of training staff to administer it was being funded by British taxpayers. Perhaps Britons felt they had obligations to Kenya, which was once a British colony, but Cameron argued there was also a hard-headed economic reason for giving foreign aid. If wealthy countries had put a fraction of current military spending into helping Afghanistan develop 20 years earlier, much conflict might have been averted. But he asserted that the main reason for giving foreign aid was a strong belief in global equity; maintaining foreign aid was simply the right thing to do. Despite pressure to cut the foreign aid budget, at the time of writing in 2018 Theresa May's UK Government has honoured David Cameron's 2015 legislative commitment to contribute 0.7% of national income to overseas aid, a target set by the WHO. Sadly in 2018 Australia's foreign aid was cut to an all-time low of 0.23% of gross national income. The US has spent less than 0.2% annually since 2015. In contrast in 2015, Sweden (1.4%), Norway (1.05%) Luxembourg (0.93%), Denmark (0.85%) and the Netherlands (0.76%) were the five most generous nations, followed by the UK.

In these days when rich governments like Australia and the United States worry about domestic spending and continually reduce foreign aid, one can only wish they would remember those ringing words of David Cameron and refuse to balance their books on the backs of the poor.

Vaccines for the poor

Existing vaccines target diseases that affect children all over the globe. However, some infections are largely confined to developing countries.

One group of infections that falls into this category is mosquito-borne diseases, such as malaria (caused by malarial parasites) and dengue fever (caused by dengue viruses). The mosquitoes that carry these organisms do not survive in temperate climates, so the infections are virtually confined to developing countries in the tropics. The lack of effective vaccines against these organisms may be caused by the fact that it is too difficult to make them, or the fact that not enough money and effort are being put into doing so.

In 2010, Paul Wilson, a scientist and economist from Columbia University working on global health policy, prepared a report for Oxfam on vaccine access for developing countries. He wrote:

Vaccine research and development is dominated by
the paradigm of multinational pharmaceutical/vaccine

companies charging high prices for products tailored to wealthy markets. Companies argue that high prices are needed to recoup research and development costs. This model distorts research and development priorities such that companies are not necessarily developing products to tackle the greatest global medical needs and are not producing products that are adapted to the particular needs of developing countries.

One vaccine whose development was delayed for many years because of a lack of will and the improbability of a return on investment was meningococcal A vaccine. The meningococcal A bacterium has a polysaccharide (sugar) outer coating similar to meningococcal C. A vaccine against meningococcal C was developed during the 1990s and introduced routinely in the United Kingdom in 1999. The vaccine is over 90% effective and has since been introduced in many other countries.

It would have been relatively easy to develop a similar vaccine for meningococcal A infection, but this infection occurs almost exclusively in poor African countries. With no financial incentive, no vaccine company was willing to develop a vaccine. Yet the devastation wreaked by meningococcal A infection dwarfed any of the problems caused by meningococcal C infection. Every 7 to 14 years, deadly epidemics of meningococcal A infection sweep across 26 countries in the so-called 'meningitis belt' of sub-Saharan Africa, from Senegal to Somalia. Thousands of children and young adults develop meningitis or bloodstream infection as a result. The worst recorded epidemic in 1997 infected an estimated 250,000 people and killed 25,000 children and young adults.

The WHO came up with a novel solution. It developed a partnership with an international not-for-profit health organisation called PATH (previously the Program for Appropriate Technology in Health) to make a meningococcal A vaccine. In 2001, the WHO set up the Meningitis Vaccine Project, which was funded for 10 years with a US$70 million grant from the Bill and Melinda Gates Foundation. The vaccine MenAfriVac was developed within a few years at a fraction of the usual cost by a Dutch biotech company, SynCo Bio Partners, in collaboration with the Center for Biologics Evaluation and Research at the United States Food and Drug Administration. Manufacture was then transferred to the Serum Institute of India. The vaccine was licensed in India in 2009 and became available for use in Africa in 2010. The final price was a remarkably low 50 cents a dose.

Vaccination campaigns were introduced from 2010 in the African countries at highest risk: Niger, Mali and Burkina Faso. In 2011, about 1.8 million people aged 1 to 29 years in Chad were immunised with a single dose of MenAfriVac during a 10-day vaccination campaign. Subsequently, the vaccine successfully prevented infection in those who had received it, while infections continued unabated in unvaccinated people.

Gavi has bought 235 million doses of the vaccine to date. It has been found to be 94% effective. In 2015, there were no cases of meningococcal A infection reported in the 16 countries that used MenAfriVac in mass vaccination campaigns. By the end of 2016, six years after its introduction, over 260 million people in Africa had been vaccinated with MenAfriVac. Ghana and Sudan included MenAfriVac in their routine immunisation schedule in 2016, the first two countries to do so.

MenAfriVac is the first ever vaccine developed specifically for the poor. It gives hope that in the future we will continue to find innovative ways to reduce inequities in health.

Reaching the needy

In 1974, when the WHO launched its Expanded Programme on Immunization, fewer than 5 million of the world's 100 million children under five were fully vaccinated against diphtheria, tetanus and pertussis. By 1990, just over a quarter of a century later, 76% of the children in the world had received the requisite three doses of DTP vaccine and 73% had received measles vaccine.

In 2016, the proportion of the world's 116.5 million children under five immunised with three doses of DTP had reached 86%. That year, 85% of the world's children received at least one dose of measles vaccine and the same proportion, 85%, received three doses of polio vaccine. The good news is that polio has been eliminated from almost all countries, and that the number of children immunised against some of the most vaccine-preventable diseases has risen from below 5 million to 100 million in less than half a century. That is formidable progress.

The bad news is that in the same year, 2016, almost 20 million children in the world did *not* receive routine immunisations such as DTP vaccine. Over half of these children (60%) live in just 10 countries: Angola, Brazil, Congo, Ethiopia, India, Indonesia, Iraq, Nigeria, Pakistan and South Africa. Some children miss out on immunisations because of war, some because of poverty and isolation.

We humans somehow worked out how to eradicate smallpox. We have almost eradicated polio. Surely it is not beyond our wit to find ways to get vaccines to those children who currently do not get them. To do so, and to sustain it, we will need to persuade developing countries that immunisations are essential for their population's health, and thus they must devote adequate resources to buying and delivering vaccines. The poorest developing countries that truly cannot afford it will need global organisations like the WHO and the United Nations and philanthropic organisations like the Bill and Melinda Gates Foundation to help out.

Former South African president Nelson Mandela memorably said: 'There can be no keener revelation of a society's soul than the way in which it treats its children.' We are talking about children, the world's capital.

CHAPTER 15

Immunisation into the future

The English satirical comedy team Monty Python once made a skit about a children's television program called 'How to Rid the World of All Known Diseases'. In the skit, one of the presenters, Jackie, breathlessly suggests the answer is to become a doctor, find a marvellous cure for something, tell the medical profession what to do and make sure they get everything right 'so there'll never be any diseases ever again'. Jolly good show.

Actually, Jackie should have been looking for a vaccine to prevent all known diseases, not a cure. Preventing a disease is much more powerful than trying to cure an ill patient.

We may contemplate the future of immunisation with excitement or apprehension or perhaps a bit of both. Excitement, because there are debilitating conditions, infectious and non-infectious, that can blight our lives and those of our loved ones, for which safe and effective vaccines would undoubtedly benefit us. Apprehension, because increasing technology scares many of us in a *Brave New World* sort of way.

The past and present of immunisation have been and are fascinating. Like all human activities, there have been bad aspects as well as good, but the overwhelming conclusion is that immunisations have been incredibly important in saving lives, preventing crippling and ruinous illnesses and improving people's quality of life. We have every reason to believe that immunisation will continue in the future to be overwhelmingly beneficial to humans.

The state of the world's health

The top 10 causes of death in the world in 2015 according to the WHO were coronary artery disease, stroke, lower respiratory tract infections, chronic obstructive pulmonary disease, lung cancer, diabetes mellitus, dementias including Alzheimer's disease, diarrhoeal diseases, tuberculosis and road traffic accidents.

Sir Macfarlane Burnet might have been more than a trifle premature in announcing 'the virtual elimination of the infectious disease' in 1962, but 100 years ago the top 10 would have included *seven* infectious diseases, not three – tuberculosis, malaria, influenza, pneumonia, gastroenteritis, diphtheria and smallpox – and infections would have caused well over half of all deaths.

Immunisation has made a huge difference. Nevertheless, we could still save many more lives simply through better use of existing vaccines. Increased access to existing pneumococcus and influenza vaccines would reduce by about half the 3.2 million deaths caused each year by lower respiratory tract infections (pneumonia), and improved access to rotavirus vaccines would prevent about 200,000 of the 1.4 million deaths annually due to diarrhoeal diseases (gastroenteritis).

These goals could be achieved by improving delivery of vaccines to the world's poorest people. As we heard in the last chapter, this would require better funding through increased philanthropy, more foreign aid and greater investment in health by poor countries.

At present both rich and poor countries spend huge amounts on weapons and armies that could, if governments only agreed on how to do so, be diverted to health and education. Surely it is not being too naïve to suggest that we should all strive to convince governments worldwide that increased spending on health and education would be money well invested, and that a strategy that promotes health at the cost of arms would also help reduce the need for those very weapons.

Vaccine wish list

Vaccine experts sometimes dream of all the diseases they could prevent through immunisation if they could just make the right vaccines, or even a single one that would prevent many diseases.

1. Malaria and HIV

These two very different diseases have dominated the vaccine wish list for the last 30 years. The organisms that cause them share the characteristic of flying beneath the radar to evade the human immune system.

Malaria is caused by a parasite transmitted by mosquitoes; HIV/AIDS is caused by a virus. They both cause chronic infection in people who often remain relatively healthy, yet can transmit the infection to others. Malaria is transmitted by the bite of an infected mosquito – but the mosquito has to bite an infected human to become infected. HIV infection can be transmitted sexually, of course, but also from an infected mother to her infant at birth or through breastfeeding. HIV is carried in the bloodstream and is also transmissible through infected blood products, such as donated blood or the blood-clotting protein Factor VIII, which infected many haemophiliacs before HIV was recognised.

Both these diseases evade our immune system in different ways, but both do so using stealth.

The malaria parasite causes disease by parasitising human red blood cells. The nastiest of the different malaria parasites, *Plasmodium falciparum*, avoids detection by switching a critical protein on and off, a bit like turning traffic lights on and off. The dangerous time for the parasite is when it is moving in the bloodstream between red blood cells, when it can be susceptible to the human immune system. By switching off the protein, the parasite becomes invisible. Once inside a red cell, it switches the protein on again, beds down and replicates. It's not exactly reds under the bed – more like an invisibility cloak.

The human immunodeficiency virus, which causes HIV infection, replicates at an enormous rate, and produces mutations that alter the way the host immune system views virus-infected cells. One mechanism is to cover HIV-infected cells with human proteins. This too has been described as using the proteins like an invisibility cloak.

Scientists have tried for many years – with really very limited success – to develop vaccines against malaria. Some vaccines have been able to prevent a proportion of cases, but no specific malaria vaccine has yet been marketed.

Fortunately, the WHO and others have had success in using medicines and innovative measures like insecticide-impregnated bed nets to reduce the global burden of malaria. The number of cases of severe malaria worldwide fell by 29% between 2010 and 2015, and although malaria still killed an estimated 429,000 people in 2015, it used to kill over a million each year.

While *Plasmodium falciparum* has had millennia to evolve mechanisms to evade the human immune system, HIV has developed the same ability despite having only recently emerged.

It is likely that HIV has only been infecting humans for 100 years at most. AIDS, the most severe illness caused by HIV, was first recognised in 1981, and HIV was identified as the source in 1983.

Scientists assured the public they would be able to develop an effective HIV vaccine rapidly. But their optimism was unfounded. Live attenuated HIV vaccines have been pretty much ruled out by the possibility that they will accidentally cause HIV infection.

Tantalus is a mythological Greek character who stole ambrosia and nectar from the gods. He was condemned to stand forever in a pool of water beneath a fruit tree with low-hanging branches. Every time he tried to grab the fruit, it eluded his grasp. When he went to drink the water in the pool, it always receded. Tantalus was tantalised to punish him for his hubris.

In medicine we talk of low-hanging fruit as something that feels as if it is almost within our grasp. Renowned immunologist Gordon Ada gave many talks on progress towards an HIV vaccine. He told me that in every talk he gave over many years, he found himself saying that the discovery was 10 years away.

Maybe we are being punished by the gods for our hubris in thinking we would find an HIV vaccine so easily.

Fortunately, as with malaria, we have made huge strides in controlling HIV without vaccines, mainly through developing highly effective medicines. When they are used optimally, a person with HIV has a life expectancy no different from that of an uninfected person.

There are problems in getting the drugs to people in poor countries, however. In 2015, HIV still killed 1.1 million people. The good news is that this is half as many as in 2005, and that HIV has now dropped out of the top 10 causes of death in the world. The bad news is that three-quarters of the deaths in 2015 were in Africa, where HIV is still the leading cause of death.

At present we are certainly making some progress towards controlling malaria and HIV, but vaccines would have the potential to save many more lives.

2. Dementia vaccines

As the population ages, the two big concerns for the elderly are their bodies and their brains. We have surgical operations, such as hip replacements, to postpone some of the ravages of skeletal deterioration. What we dream of is something that would prevent dementia. What we dread is that our nearest and dearest will suffer from the condition, or that we ourselves will.

Dementias are diseases that cause impaired memory and thinking. Alzheimer's disease is perhaps the best known, but there are several others. British writer Terry Pratchett made light of his own dementia when he wrote: 'It is possible to live well with dementia and write best sellers like wot I do.' But he also railed over being an author who lost his facility with words, and he died at just 66.

In 2015, over 1.5 million people in the world died from a form of dementia. In 2015, dementias featured for the first time among the WHO's top 10 causes of death, coming in at number seven.

Clearly, the rise of dementia is partly because we are living longer. However, we do not know the cause and have no effective treatment. There is some evidence that 'clean living' – avoiding drugs, excessive alcohol and tobacco, and using your brain a lot – are preventative to a certain extent. There is also evidence that dementia can run in families.

Scientists have actually made dementia vaccines, but they are being tested on people who already have dementia, whereas the ideal approach would be to vaccinate to *prevent* the disease.

There is a good reason why these vaccines are only being given to dementia sufferers. The brains of people suffering from Alzheimer's disease have two characteristics: the accumulation of a protein called amyloid-beta (also written as amyloid-β or Aβ), and an excess of neurofibrillary tangles. 'Neurofibrillary tangles' seems like a poignant description of the state of the brains in which they are found. They are actually accumulations of tau protein (named after the Greek letter τ).

Both amyloid and tau proteins occur naturally, but accumulate to excess in Alzheimer's patients. And there's the rub. If the proteins occur naturally, would a vaccine against the proteins cause harm if given to someone who is at risk of dementia but is currently normal?

Scientists have developed vaccines against both amyloid-β and tau proteins and have studied them in animals and in humans with Alzheimer's disease. The vaccines did not cause demonstrable harm, but neither did the subjects show any improvement in cognitive function.

It would be naïvely optimistic to think that a therapeutic vaccine could reverse brain damage in people with dementia, although the idea is not impossible. Perhaps in future we will be able to identify – for example, through genetic testing – people at high risk who might be candidates for a preventative vaccine.

New modes of delivery

Some of people's resistance to immunisation is based on the invasive nature of injecting foreign substances. Less invasive routes have the potential to deliver vaccines much more cheaply, easily and painlessly.

1. Oral vaccines

We already use oral vaccines containing attenuated strains against polio and rotavirus. Both of these are gut viruses that enter the body through the intestine. Oral vaccines cannot be used for respiratory viruses, because they are destroyed by the acid in our stomachs. Other potential oral vaccines have remained just out of the reach of some of our most innovative and inventive scientists.

In Chapter 8, on vaccines and cancer, we learned about two West Australian scientists, Barry Marshall and Robin Warren, and their discovery of the bacterium *Helicobacter pylori*. Although there is no vaccine against *Helicobacter pylori* on the market, in 2005 a Chinese group published a study showing that an oral artificial (not live) vaccine protected 72% of children against *Helicobacter pylori* infection. An effective oral vaccine would have the potential to prevent cancer of the stomach and save thousands of people from a painful, miserable death.

Edible vaccines are vaccines produced in genetically modified plants that can be eaten. The name was coined by American molecular biologist Charles Arntzen in 1990. An edible vaccine is developed by finding a way of inserting a gene coding into a plant.

Our current hepatitis B vaccines use the protein on the outside of the virus called the surface antigen, which has the genetic code HBsAg. Arntzen and other researchers showed in 1992 that they could grow tobacco plants that incorporated the HBsAg gene. The plants were not edible, but it was proof of the concept of plant-derived vaccines.

Arntzen and others have gone on to develop edible hepatitis B vaccines by inserting the HBsAg gene into tomatoes, bananas, rice and algae. (An edible vaccine is not necessarily palatable, although obviously it will be better tolerated if it tastes good.) Other plants used to make edible vaccines are alfalfa, apples, carrots, lettuce, maize, papaya, potatoes, quinoa and soy beans. The hope was that they would be cheap to produce – at least after the initial cost of developing the vaccine – as well as cheap to deliver and easy to administer. I know a vaccine scientist who dropped everything in the early 1990s and devoted the rest of his career to trying to grow hepatitis B vaccine in potatoes.

Sadly, initial excitement at the prospect of edible vaccines has been tempered by practical issues. The public has often expressed concern about genetically modified crops with regard to human safety, environmental conservation and the risks of 'tampering with nature'; genetically modified edible vaccines raise similar biosafety issues. There are concerns about traces of pesticides.

Allergy to plants is another possible problem. Ensuring the correct dose can be difficult. The cost of preserving and delivering edible vaccines makes them more expensive than hoped. Vaccines grown in plants that are unpalatable when raw, such as potatoes, need to remain active after cooking.

Despite the initial excitement, there are no edible vaccines currently licensed for use in humans. A United States vaccine grown in tobacco cells is available to protect against Newcastle disease, which can decimate poultry. Researchers have made some headway towards developing an edible vaccine against Ebola virus, and the ideal would be to develop an edible Ebola vaccine that not only protected against Ebola but also had nutritional value.

The potential for edible vaccines is huge, but the difficulties remain considerable. Nevertheless, it is possible that safe, effective edible vaccines will be available in the foreseeable future.

2. Nasal vaccines

A family is a unit composed not only of children but of men, women, an occasional animal and the common cold.

Ogden Nash, poet (1902–1971)

Nasal vaccines target cells in the lining of the nose (nasal mucosa), so they have the advantage of stimulating nasal immunity as well as being generally better tolerated than injected vaccines. Researchers have tried for decades to develop nasal vaccines against the respiratory viruses that cause colds and more severe diseases.

The most obvious candidate is influenza. A live attenuated nasal influenza vaccine called FluMist was developed by United

States researchers as a nasal spray in the 1990s. It has been used as an alternative to injected influenza vaccine in the United States since 2003, although it has not yet been marketed in Australia.

Respiratory syncytial virus (RSV) is a virus found in almost every country in the world. (We looked at it in the section on pneumonia back in Chapter 7.) It is most virulent when it infects infants, in whom it can cause a life-threatening respiratory infection called bronchiolitis. No one has succeeded in developing a safe, injectable RSV vaccine. Attempts to develop a nasal live attenuated RSV vaccine for infants have been hampered by the tension between causing a low-grade infection that does not stimulate enough immunity, and causing a high-grade infection that results in worrying nasal congestion. The same problem has hampered the development of an effective nasal vaccine against parainfluenza viruses, which can cause croup. Nevertheless, researchers are still hopeful of developing safe, effective nasal vaccines against RSV and parainfluenza viruses that will be easy to deliver and will make a huge difference to children's health.

3. Skin vaccines

The skin should be an ideal site for vaccine delivery because it contains branching cells called dendritic cells that are involved in the immune response.

Jet injectors can deliver vaccines into the skin under pressure, without the need for a needle. They have been used to give inactivated polio vaccine to young children in Cuba and BCG vaccine to adults and newborns in South Africa. The only study that has compared pain from jet injectors with pain from conventional immunisation found, however, that the jet injectors were more painful than intramuscular injections in adults. Given that one reason for using needle-free vaccine delivery is to reduce pain, this is an obvious drawback.

One advantage of jet injectors is that they can be used for multiple vaccinations, which saves time and money. However, strict infection control precautions must be observed to prevent transmission of organisms from person to person. An outbreak of hepatitis B infection occurred between 1984 and 1985 in a weight-reduction clinic that gave hormones using jet injectors. The pressing need (no pun intended) to avoid such outbreaks is a major consideration in deciding whether to use jet injectors in immunisation programs.

Professor Mark Kendall is a bioengineer from the University of Queensland who has devoted his career to developing a technology called the nanopatch. Similar to a Band-Aid (sticking plaster), the nanopatch is covered with thousands of minuscule needles coated with vaccine. When you apply the nanopatch it immunises you painlessly through your skin.

This may sound easy, but the technology required to deliver the right amount of vaccine is highly complex. Mark Kendall's team has published the results of successful experiments in mice, and is now carrying out early human studies. However, teams in other countries, including the United States, are competing to produce the best system of microneedles, and have developed techniques known colourfully as 'poke and flow', 'poke and patch', 'poke and release' and 'coat and poke'.

In 2017, a research team from Emory University, Alabama, beat Mark Kendall in publishing the first human study. They used sticking-plaster-sized patches containing only 100 needles, not the thousands in Kendall's nanopatch, and compared the use of a single microneedle patch with the usual intramuscular injection in delivering influenza vaccine to 100 adults, with 50 using a patch and 50 receiving an intramuscular injection.

A patch was stuck onto the back of each volunteer's hand, or study participants could apply it themselves; it could then be peeled away after a few days and discarded. Within minutes of being inserted into the skin, the patch dissolved, releasing the vaccine. The main adverse effect was itch and localised redness for two to three days, but 48 of the 50 volunteers said the patch was painless, and 70% said they greatly preferred the patch to an intramuscular injection.

The patches are stable for at least one year at 40°C, which is useful for maintaining the cold chain. Another advantage is that the patch avoids the need to dispose of sharp needles. This new approach could improve influenza immunisation coverage by appealing to people who dislike needles, and should reduce the cost of giving immunisations.

The immunisation saga started centuries ago, when material from smallpox sores was scratched crudely into people's arms in China and Turkey, in a technique that came to be called variolation. We have now come almost full circle: patches also induce an immune response by delivering foreign material directly into the skin, albeit with greater sophistication. What charming irony – but how indicative too of the technological leaps we have achieved within a relatively short period of human history.

Conclusion

In 1720 there were no vaccines. By 1820, smallpox vaccine was available for routine use, and rabies vaccine could be given to people bitten by a rabid animal. By 1920, countries like the United States, the United Kingdom and Australia were starting to give diphtheria vaccine. In 2020, young children in many countries will routinely receive vaccines against diphtheria, tetanus, pertussis, polio, Hib, hepatitis B, rotavirus, measles, mumps, rubella, varicella, meningococcus and pneumococcus. Schoolchildren will be immunised against human papillomavirus infection and cervical cancer will be on the way out. Infants in developing countries will be routinely immunised against tuberculosis. Vaccines against other diseases like yellow fever and hepatitis A will be used widely in areas where they are most needed. New vaccines will be developed against other infectious scourges.

What remarkable progress we have made.

The history of immunisation is full of enchantment and excitement and extraordinary drama, and the future looks equally entrancing. The story of vaccines and their delivery has featured many famous scientists and unsung heroes who risked and sometimes lost their lives, as well as its fair share of villains.

Wonderful tales such as the delivery of meningococcal A vaccine in Africa and the elimination of polio from the world are still emerging in the present day. We should be optimistic that, in the future, immunisation will continue to yield exciting and uplifting examples of human endeavour and achievement.

We may not yet have prevented all known diseases, but immunisation has made and will continue to make a massive difference to people's lives. The past, present and future of immunisation constitute surely one of the greatest of all human stories.

Endnotes

CHAPTER 1: Our deadliest foes

Willie Lincoln: The death of Willie Lincoln. *Abraham Lincoln Online*, www.abrahamlincolnonline.org/lincoln/education/williedeath.htm.

Plague of Athens: Finley MI. *The Greek Historians: The Essence of Herodotus, Thucydides, Xenophon, Polybius.* Harmondsworth: Penguin Books, 1977; The plague. *Livius*, www.livius.org/sources/content/thucydides/the-plague/.

Genetic make-up of humans and viruses: Willyard C. New human gene tally reignites debate. *Nature* 2018; 558: 354–5, www.nature.com/articles/d41586–018–05462-w; Bouvier NM, Palese P. The biology of influenza viruses. *Vaccine* 2008; 26 (Suppl 4): D49–53, www.ncbi.nlm.nih.gov/pmc/articles/PMC3074182/.

European colonisation of the Americas: Diamond J. *Guns, Germs and Steel: The Fate of Human Societies.* New York: WW Norton & Co, 1997 (winner of the Pulitzer Prize).

1918 influenza pandemic: Spinney L. *Pale Rider: The Spanish Flu of 1918 and How It Changed the World.* London: Vintage, 2017; Porter KA. *Pale Horse, Pale Rider.* London: Penguin Classics, 2011; Persico JE. The great swine flu epidemic of 1918. *American Heritage* 1976; 27: 4, www.americanheritage.com/content/greats-wine-flu-epidemic-1918.

Olivia Dahl: Death of Olivia. *Roald Dahl*, www.roalddahl.com/roald-dahl/timeline/1960s/november-1962.

Herd immunity: Reichert TA et al. The Japanese experience with vaccinating schoolchildren against influenza. *N Engl J Med* 2001; 344: 889–96, www.nejm.org/doi/full/10.1056/NEJM200103223441204; Hardin G. The tragedy of the commons. *Science* 1968; 162: 1243–8, www.geo.mtu.edu/~asmayer/rural_sustain/governance/Hardin%201968.pdf; Browne K. Measles, vaccination, and the tragedy of the commons. *The Hastings Center*, 25 February 2015, www.thehastingscenter.org/measles-vaccination-and-the-tragedy-of-the-commons/.

Whooping cough vaccine and encephalopathy: Baker JP. The pertussis vaccine controversy in Great Britain, 1974–1986. *Vaccine* 2003; 21: 4003–10.

MMR vaccine and autism: Wakefield AJ, Murch SH, Anthony A et al. Ileal lymphoid nodular hyperplasia, non-specific colitis, and pervasive developmental disorder in children (retracted). *Lancet* 1998; 351: 637–41; Deer B. How the case against the MMR vaccine was fixed. *BMJ* 2011; 342: c5347, www.bmj.com/content/342/bmj.c5347; Deer B. How the vaccine crisis was meant to make money. *BMJ* 2011; 342: c5258, www.bmj.com/content/342/bmj.c5258.full; Godlee F et al. Wakefield's article linking MMR vaccine and autism was fraudulent. *BMJ* 2011; 342: c7452, www.bmj.com/content/342/bmj.c7452.

ABC documentary: Chapman S. Tilting at the immunisation windmill. BMJ 1997; 314: 1641; https://www.bmj.com/content/314/7095/1641.15.full

CHAPTER 2: Smallpox, the speckled monster

History of smallpox: Hopkins DR. *Princes and Peasants: Smallpox in History*. Chicago: University of Chicago Press, 1983.

Plague of Galen: Littmann RJ, Littmann ML. Galen and the Antonine plague. *Am J Philology* 1973; 94: 243–55.

Elizabeth I: Whitelock A. *Elizabeth's Bedfellows: An Intimate History of the Queen's Court*. London: Bloomsbury Press, 2013; Hume MAS (ed). *Calendar of Letters and State Papers Relating to English Affairs: Volume 1*. Cambridge: Cambridge Library Collection, 1983.

Mortality rates in 18th and early 19th centuries: Davenport R, Schwarz L, Boulton, J. The decline of adult smallpox in eighteenth-century

London. *Econ Hist Rev* 20011; 64 (4): 1289–1314; https://www.ncbi.
nlm.nih.gov/pmc/articles/PMC4373148/.

Turlough O'Carolan: O'Sullivan D. *Carolan: The Life Times and Music of an
Irish Harper.* Cork: Ossian Publications, 2001.

French and Indian War: d'Errico P. Jeffery Amherst and smallpox blankets.
U Mass Amherst, people.umass.edu/derrico/amherst/lord_jeff.html.

Sydney outbreak: The origin of the smallpox outbreak in Sydney in 1789.
Treaty Republic, 2008, treatyrepublic.net/node/651; Warren C. Was
Sydney's smallpox outbreak of 1789 an act of biological warfare
against Aboriginal tribes? *Ockham's Razor,* 17 April 2014, www.abc.
net.au/radionational/programs/ockhamsrazor/was-sydneys-smallpox-
outbreak-an-act-of-biological-warfare/5395050; Tench W. *A Complete
Account of the Settlement at Port Jackson.* Adelaide: University of
Adelaide Library, ebooks.adelaide.edu.au/t/tench/watkin/settlement/
chapter4.html; Moorehad A. *The Fatal Impact: An Account of the
Invasion of the South Pacific,* 1767–1840. Ringwood, Victoria,
Australia: Penguin Books Ltd, 1966.

Lord Macaulay: Potter P. The fragrance of the heifer's breath. *Emerging
Infectious Diseases* 2011; 17: 763–4.

History of variolation: Behbehani A. The smallpox story: life and death of an
old disease. *Microbiol Rev* 1983; 47: 455–509, www.ncbi.nlm.nih.gov/
pmc/articles/PMC281588/pdf/microrev00019–0005.pdf.

Emanuele Timoni: Timoni E. An account, or history, of the procuring of
the smallpox by incision or inoculation, as it has for some time been
practised at Constantinople. *Philosophical Transactions of the Royal
Society* 1714–1716; 29: 72–82.

Lady Mary Wortley Montagu: Grundy I. Montagu, Lady Mary Wortley.
Oxford Dictionary of National Biography. Oxford: Oxford University
Press, 2004, dx.doi.org/10.1093/ref:odnb/19029.

Benjamin Franklin: Franklin B. *The Autobiography of Benjamin Franklin.*
New York: Simon & Schuster, 2004.

John Adams: Gelles EB. *Abigail and John: Portrait of a Marriage.* New
York: William Morrow, 2009; Adams' Argument for the defense: 3–4
December 1770. *Founders Online,* founders.archives.gov/documents/
Adams/05–03–02–0001–0004–0016.

Edward Jenner: Baxby D. Jenner, Edward. *Oxford Dictionary of National Biography*. Oxford: Oxford University Press, www.oxforddnb. com/view/10.1093/ref:odnb/9780198614128.001.0001/odnb-9780198614128-e-14749; Jenner E. Observations on the natural history of the cuckoo. By Mr Edward Jenner. In a letter to John Hunter, Esq FRS. *Philosophical Transactions of the Royal Society of London (1776–1886)* 1 January 1788; 78: 219–37, archive.org/details/philtrans06624558. Edward Jenner. *Brought to life*, Science Museum; http://broughttolife.sciencemuseum.org.uk/broughttolife/people/edwardjenner

Benjamin Jesty: Pead PJ. Benjamin Jesty: new light in the dawn of immunisation. *Lancet* 2003; 362: 2104–9.

Catherine the Great: Ben-Menahem A. *Historical Encyclopedia of Natural and Mathematical Sciences*. New York: Springer, 2009.

John Savage: Weston KM, Gallagher WC, Branley JM. Smallpox vaccination, colonial Sydney and serendipity. *Med J Aust* 2014; 200: 295–7, www.mja.com.au/system/files/issues/200_05_170314/wes11021_fm.pdf.

Dr Alex Cook: Cook A. The preservation of the vaccine lymph. *Sydney Morning Herald*, 6 March 1843.

1841 vaccine sample: Forwarding vaccine virus. NSW Government State Archives & Records: Colonial Secretary; NRS 905, Main series of letters received, 1841 Medical (4/2531.4). Letter No. 41/5095 Deputy Inspector General of Hospitals (Dr Thompson), registered 21 May 1841; Vaccine sample from 1841 found in the archives. NSW Government State Archives & Records, www.records.nsw. gov.au/archives/collections-and-research/guides-and-indexes/stories/vaccine-sample-1841-found-the-archives; Weston KM, Gallagher WC, Branley JM. Smallpox vaccination, colonial Sydney and serendipity. *Med J Aust* 2014; 200: 295–7, www.mja.com.au/system/files/issues/200_05_170314/wes11021_fm.pdf.

Anti-vaccination protests: History of anti-vaccination movements. *The History of Vaccines*, www.historyofvaccines.org/content/articles/history-anti-vaccination-movements; Crutch D (ed). *Lewis Carroll: Three Letters on Anti-vaccination (1877)*. London: Lewis Carroll Society, 1976; Rolleston JD. The smallpox pandemic of 1870–1874. *Proc Roy Soc Med* 1933; 27: 177–92, journals.sagepub.com/doi/

pdf/10.1177/003591573302700245; Mariner WK et al. *Jacobson v Massachusetts*: it's not your great-great-grandfather's public health law. *Am J Public Health* 2005; 95: 4: 581–90, www.ncbi.nlm.nih.gov/pmc/articles/PMC1449224/.

Smallpox eradication: Foege WH. *House on Fire: The Fight to Eradicate Smallpox*. Berkeley: University of California Press, 2011; Fenner F, Henderson DA, Arita I, Jezek Z, Ladnyi D. *Smallpox and Its Eradication (History of International Public Health, No 6)*. Geneva: World Health Organization, 1988.

DA Henderson: Dennis, B. DA Henderson helped eradicate smallpox. He also used to keep it in his fridge. Washington Post, 21 August 2016.

Rhondda Valley outbreak: 1962 South Wales smallpox outbreak memories recorded. *BBC News*, 12 June 2012, www.bbc.com/news/uk-wales-18365385; Mansworth S. Deadly disease; analysis: survivors of the 1962 South Wales smallpox outbreak have helped to paint a terrifying portrait of how the UK would cope with a bio-terrorist attack. *Free Library* 2002, www.thefreelibrary.com/DEADLY+DISEASE%3B+Analys is%3A+Survivors+of+the+1962+South+Wales+smallpox ... -a082591810.

CHAPTER 3: The flawed genius of Louis Pasteur

Life of Louis Pasteur: Debré P. Forster E (transl). *Louis Pasteur*. Baltimore: JHU Press, 2000; Ligon BL. Biography: Louis Pasteur: a controversial figure. *Seminars in Pediatric Infectious Disease* 2002; 13: 134–41, www.sciencedirect.com/science/article/pii/S1045187002500595; Vallery-Redot R, Devonshire R (transl). *The Life of Pasteur*. Vol 2. New York: Doubleday, 1923, archive.org/stream/lifeofpasteur02vall/lifeofpasteur02vall_djvu.txt.

Rabies: Finnegan CJ et al. Rabies in North America and Europe. *J Roy Soc Med* 2002; 95: 9–13, www.ncbi.nlm.nih.gov/pmc/articles/PMC1279140/.

Emile Roux: Delaunay A. Roux, Pierre Paul Emile. *Complete Dictionary of Scientific Biography*. New York: Charles Scribner's Sons, 2008.

Louis Pasteur's notebooks: Geison GL. *The Private Science of Louis Pasteur*. Princeton: Princeton University Press, 1995; Fee E. Book review: *The Private Science of Louis Pasteur*. NEJM 1995; 333: 8: 84–5, www.nejm.org/doi/pdf/10.1056/NEJM199509283331321.

CHAPTER 4: The end of polio

FDR: Black C. *Franklin Delano Roosevelt: Champion of Freedom.*
Cambridge, Massachusetts: Public Affairs, 2003; Coker JW. *Franklin
D Roosevelt: A Biography.* Westport, Connecticut: Greenwood
Press, 2005; Beckman M. Did FDR have Guillain-Barré? *Science,*
31 October 2003, www.sciencemag.org/news/2003/10/did-fdr-have-
guillain-barr.

Polio victims: Marshall A. *I Can Jump Puddles.* Melbourne: FW Cheshire,
1955; Offit P. *The Cutter Incident: How America's First Polio Vaccine
Led to the Growing Vaccine Crisis.* New Haven: Yale University Press,
2005; Roth P. *Nemesis.* Boston: Houghton Mifflin Harcourt, 2010.

Sister Kenny: National Library of Australia. Kenny, Elizabeth (1880–1952),
trove.nla.gov.au/people/493848?c=people; Pearn J. The Sylvia
stretcher: a perspective of Sister Elizabeth Kenny's contribution to
the first-aid management of injured patients. *Med J Aust* 1988; 149:
636–8; Kenny E. *Infantile Paralysis and Cerebral Diplegia: Method of
Restoration of Function.* Sydney: Angus & Robertson, 1937.

Dr Morris Fishbein: Cohn V. *Sister Kenny: The Woman Who Challenged the
Doctors.* Minneapolis, University of Minnesota Press, 1976.

Albert Sabin and Jonas Salk: Norkin LC. Jonas Salk and Albert Sabin:
One of the great rivalries of medical science. *Virology: Molecular
Biology and Pathogenesis,* 27 March 2014, norkinvirology.wordpress.
com/2014/03/27/jonas-salk-and-albert-sabin-one-of-the-great-
rivalries-of-medical-science/; Oshinsky DM. *Polio: An American
Story.* Oxford: Oxford University Press, 2006.

Polio in India: John JT, Vasitha VM. Eradicating poliomyelitis: India's
journey from hyperendemic to polio-free status. *Indian J Med Res*
2013; 137: 881–94.

Ciro de Quadros: Seaton D. Remembering Ciro de Quadros, vaccines
champion. *BIOtechNOW,* 6 April 2014, www.biotech-now.org/
health/2014/06/remembering-ciro-de-quadros-vaccines-champion.

Polio in Pakistan: Riaz H, RehmanA. Polio vaccination workers gunned
down in Pakistan. *Lancet Infect Dis.* 2013; 13: 120; Bhutta ZA.
What must be done about the killings of Pakistani healthcare
workers? *BMJ* 2013; 346: f280; Saleem S. Muslim scholars
fight to dispel polio vaccination myths in Pakistan. *Guardian,*

5 November 2011, www.theguardian.com/commentisfree/
belief/2011/nov/04/polio-vaccination-pakistan; www.theguardian.
com/world/pakistan+society/polio; Rasmussen SE. Polio in
Afghanistan: 'Americans bomb our children daily, why would they
care?', *Guardian*, 10 April 2017, www.theguardian.com/global-
development/2017/apr/10/polio-afghanistan-taliban-health-chief-
americans-bomb-children; Janjua H. Afghan clerics in talks with Isis
to break polio myths. *Guardian*, 27 March 2018. www.theguardian.
com/global-development/2018/mar/27/afghan-clerics-in-talks-with-
isis-to-break-polio-myths.

Polio in Nigeria: Ahmed S et al. Police officers gunned down while protecting
vaccination workers in Pakistan. *J Infect Public Health* 2017; 10: 249–
50; McNeil Jr DG. Gunmen kill Nigerian polio vaccine workers in
echo of Pakistan attacks. *New York Times*, 8 February 2013, nytimes.
com/2013/02/09/world/africa/in-nigeria-polio-vaccine-workers-are-
killed-by-gunmen.html.

'Polio endgame': Aylward B, Yamada T. The polio endgame. *N Engl
J Med* 2011; 364: 2273–5, www.nejm.org/doi/full/10.1056/
NEJMp1104329#t=article; Garon J, Patel M. The polio endgame:
rationale behind the change in immunisation. *Arch Dis Child* 2017;
102: 362–5, adc.bmj.com/content/archdischild/102/4/362.full.pdf.

CHAPTER 5: Tuberculosis, the great equaliser

TB in literature: Dickens C. *The Life and Adventures of Nicholas Nickleby.*
London: Chapman & Hall, 1839; Sontag S. *Illness as Metaphor.* New
York: Farrar, Straus & Giroux, 1978; Mukherjee S. *The Emperor of
All Maladies: A Biography of Cancer.* New York: Simon & Schuster,
2010; Keats J. *Lamia, Isabella, The Eve of St Agnes, and Other
Poems.* London: Taylor and Hessey, 1820.

Origins of TB: Chisholm R et al. Controlled fire use in early humans might
have triggered the evolutionary emergence of tuberculosis. *PNAS*
2016; 113: 9051–6, www.pnas.org/content/113/32/9051.full.pdf.

TB and fashion: www.smithsonianmag.com/science-nature/how-tuberculosis-
shaped-victorian-fashion-180959029.

Effectiveness of BCG vaccine: Mangtani P et al. Protection by BCG vaccine
against tuberculosis: a systematic review of randomized controlled

trials. *Clin Infect Dis* 2014; **58**: 470–80, academic.oup.com/cid/article-lookup/doi/10.1093/cid/cit790.

Outdated measures against TB: Le Get R. Isolation, collapsing lungs and spitting bans: three ways we used to treat TB, and still might. *The Conversation*, 15 September 2017, theconversation.com/isolation-collapsing-lungs-and-spitting-bans-three-ways-we-used-to-treat-tb-and-still-might-81685.

James Lind: White M. James Lind: the man who helped to cure scurvy with lemons. BBC News, 4 October 2016, www.bbc.com/news/uk-england-37320399.

TB statistics: Tuberculosis. *World Health Organization*, www.who.int/tb/en/;www.who.int/news-room/fact-sheets/detail/tuberculosis.

CHAPTER 6: Diptheria, the scourge of childhood

Langdon Clemens: White J. Diphtheria killed Langdon, Mark Twain's baby son. *Write to the Point!* 27 September 2013, twainstudios.com/2013/09/27/diphtheria-killed-twains-baby-son-langdon/.

Joost van Lom: Andrewes F, Bulloch W, Douglas SR, Dreyer G, Gardner AD, Fildes P, Ledingham JCG, Wolf CGL. *Diphtheria: Its Bacteriology, Pathology and Immunology.* London: Medical Research Council, 1923.

Year of strangulations: Laval E. El garotillo (difteria) en España (siglos XVI y XVII). *Revista Chilena de Infectología* 2006; **23**: 78–80; Guilfoyle PG. *Diphtheria.* New York: Chelsea House, 2009.

Pierre Bretonneau: Rolleston JD. Bretonneau: his life and work. *Proceedings of the* Royal Society *of Medicine, Section of the History of Medicine,* 1924: 18, journals.sagepub.com/doi/pdf/10.1177/003591572501801701.

Edwin Klebs and Friedrich Löffler: Gleason WS. The antitoxin treatment of diphtheria. *BMJ* 1894; **2**: 931–3, www.jstor.org/stable/20230288.

William H Park: Oliver WW. *The Man Who Lived for Tomorrow: A Biography of William Hallock Park, MD.* New York: EP Dutton, 1941.

1990s diphtheria outbreak: Vitek CR, Wharton M. Diphtheria in the former Soviet Union: reemergence of a pandemic disease. *Emerg Infect Dis* 1998; **4**: 539–50, wwwnc.cdc.gov/eid/article/4/4/98–0404_article.

Diphtheria in the United States: WHO vaccine-preventable diseases: monitoring system. 2018 global summary, *World Health Organization*, apps.who.int/immunization_monitoring/ globalsummary/incidences?c=United States.

Australian diphtheria case, January 2018: McCosker R. Cairns man dies from diphtheria. *Brisbane Times*, 8 February 2018, www. brisbanetimes.com.au/national/queensland/cairns-man-dies-from-diphtheria-20180208-p4yzo2.html.

CHAPTER 7: The golden age of immunisation

Immunisation in Australia: History of vaccination in Australia. *National Centre for Immunisation Research & Surveillance*, www.ncirs.edu.au/ provider-resources/vaccination-history/.

Edwin Smith Papyrus: van Middentrop JJ, Sanchez GM, Burridge AL. The Edwin Smith papyrus: a clinical reappraisal of the oldest known document on spinal injuries. *Eur Spine J* 2010; 19: 1815–23, www. ncbi.nlm.nih.gov/pmc/articles/PMC2989268/; jnnp.bmj.com/ content/63/6/758

Arthur Nicolaier: Schagen U. Arthur Nicolaier. *Charité Memorial Site*, 2013, gedenkort.charite.de/en/projects/people/arthur_nicolaier/.

Whooping cough: Kuchar E, Karlikowska-Skwarnik M, Han S, Nitsch-Osuch A. Pertussis: history of the disease and current prevention failure. *Adv Exp Med Biol* 2016; 934: 77–82; TEC Jr. A novel Irish cure for whooping cough and chickenpox (1898). *Pediatrics* 1978; 61: 251, pediatrics.aappublications.org/content/61/2/251; Dr Leila Denmark. Obituary. *Daily Telegraph*, 6 June 2018, www.telegraph.co.uk/news/ obituaries/medicine-obituaries/9190936/Dr-Leila-Denmark.html.

Hib: Watt JP, Wolfson LJ, O'Brien KL. Burden of disease caused by *Haemophilus influenzae* type b in children younger than 5 years: global estimates. *Lancet* 2009; 374: 903–11, www.who.int/ immunization/diseases/hib/GBD_Hib.pdf.

Hib immunisation: Haemophilus influenzae type b (Hib), *World Health Organization*, www.who.int/immunization/topics/hib/en/.

Pneumococcus immunisation: Pneumococcal disease, *World Health Organization*, www.who.int/immunization/topics/pneumococcal_ disease/en/.

Meningococcal meningitis: Patel MS. Australia's century of meningococcal disease: development and the changing ecology of an accidental pathogen. *Med J Aust* 2007; 186: 136–41.

Hepatitis B and sport: Kordi R, Wallace WA. Blood borne infections in sport: risks of transmission, methods of prevention, and recommendations for hepatitis B vaccination. *Br J Sports Med* 2004; 38: 678–84, bjsm. bmj.com/content/38/6/678#ref-23; Ringertz O, Zetterberg B. Serum hepatitis among Swedish track finders – an epidemiologic study. *N Engl J Med* 1967; 276: 540–6, www.nejm.org/doi/full/10.1056/ NEJM196703092761003; Kashiwagi S et al. An outbreak of hepatitis B in members of a high school sumo wrestling club. *JAMA* 1982; 248: 213–4, jamanetwork.com/journals/jama/fullarticle/vol/248/pg/213; Tobe K et al. Horizontal transmission of hepatitis B virus among players of an American football team. *Arch Intern Med* 2000; 160: 2541–5, jamanetwork.com/journals/jamainternalmedicine/article-abstract/485418.

Rotavirus: Immunization, vaccines and biologicals: rotavirus. *World Health Organization*, www.who.int/immunization/diseases/rotavirus/en/.

Arrival of measles in Australia: Paterson BJ, Kirk MD, Cameron AS, D'Este C, Durrheim D. Historical data and modern methods reveal insights in measles epidemiology: a retrospective closed cohort study. *BMJ Open* 2013; 3: e002033, bmjopen.bmj.com/content/3/1/e002033

Measles vaccines: Demicheli V, Rivetti A, Debalini MG, DiPietrantonj C. Vaccines for measles, mumps and rubella in children.*Cochrane Database of Systematic Reviews* 2012; 2: CD004407; Peltola H, Heinonen OP. Frequency of true adverse reactions to measles-mumps-rubella vaccine. A double-blind placebo-controlled trial in twins. *Lancet* 1986; 1: 939–42.

Measles statistics: Measles. *World Health Organization*, www.who.int/news-room/fact-sheets/detail/measles.

2014 Ohio measles outbreak: Gastañaduy PA et al. A measles outbreak in an underimmunized Amish community in Ohio. *N Engl J Med* 2016; 375: 1343–54.

Congenital rubella: Khandaker G et al. Surveillance for congenital rubella in Australia since 1993: cases reported between 2004 and 2013. *Vaccine* 2014; 32: 6746–51.

Chickenpox: Aronson J. Chickenpox. *BMJ* 2000; 321: 682, www.ncbi.nlm. nih.gov/pmc/articles/PMC1118558/; TEC Jr. A novel Irish cure for whooping cough and chicken pox (1898). *Pediatrics* 1978; 61: 251, pediatrics.aappublications.org/content/61/2/251; Ozaki T, Asano Y. Development of varicella vaccine in Japan and future prospects. *Vaccine* 2016; 34: 3427–33.

HPV vaccine: Cervical cancer statistics. *Cancer Australia*, cervical-cancer. canceraustralia.gov.au/statistics; National cancer control indicators: HPV vaccination uptake, *Cancer Australia*, ncci.canceraustralia.gov. au/prevention/hpv-vaccination-uptake/hpv-vaccination-uptake; Hall MT et al. The projected timeframe until cervical cancer elimination in Australia: a modelling study. *Lancet Public Health* 2018. Published online 2 October 2018, dx.doi.org/10.1016/S2468-2667(18)30183-X.

CHAPTER 8: Vaccines and cancer

Bob Marley: Steffens R, Johnson LK. *So Much Things to Say: The Oral History of Bob Marley.* New York: WW Norton & Co, 2017.

Snuff and cancer: Morris AD. 'Sir' John Hill, MA, MD (1706–1775): apothecary, botanist, playwright, actor, novelist, journalist. *Proc Roy Soc Med* 1960; 53: 55–60, www.ncbi.nlm.nih.gov/pmc/articles/ PMC1870866/.

Soot and cancer: Kipling D, Waldron HA. Percivall Pott and cancer scroti. *Br J Indust Med* 1975; 32: 244–50, oem.bmj.com/content/ oemed/32/3/244.full.pdf.

Hepatitis B statistics: D'Souza R, Foster GR. Diagnosis and treatment of chronic hepatitis B *J Roy Soc Med* 2004; 97: 318–21, www.ncbi.nlm. nih.gov/pmc/articles/PMC1079522/; Chang MH, Chen CJ, Lai MS et al. Universal hepatitis B vaccination in Taiwan and the incidence of hepatocellular carcinoma in children. *N Engl J Med* 1997; 336: 1855–9, www.nejm.org/doi/pdf/10.1056/NEJM199706263362602.

Baruch Blumberg: Alter H. Baruch Blumberg (1925–2011): obituary. *Nature* 2011; 473: 155, www.nature.com/articles/473155a; Schütte K et al. Prevention of hepatocellular carcinoma. *Gastrointest Tumors* 2016; 3: 37–43, www.ncbi.nlm.nih.gov/pmc/articles/PMC5040884/.

George Papanicolaou: Carmichael DE. *The Pap Smear: Life of George N Papanicolaou.* Springfield, Illinois: Charles C Thomas, 1973;

Papanicolaou G. New cancer diagnosis. *CA Cancer J Clin* 1973; 23: 174–9 (presented at the Third Race Betterment Conference, Battle Creek, Michigan, 2 to 6 January 1928, and first published in the proceedings of the conference).

Harald zur Hausen: Gasparini R, Panatto D. Cervical cancer: from Hippocrates through Rigoni-Stern to zur Hausen. *Vaccine* 2009; 27(Suppl 1): A4–A5.

Suzanne Garland: Garland SM et al. Quadrivalent vaccine against human papillomavirus to prevent anogenital diseases. *N Engl J Med* 2007; 356: 1928–43, www.nejm.org/doi/pdf/10.1056/NEJMoa061760.

Cost of HPV vaccines: Clendinen C et al. Manufacturing costs of HPV vaccines for developing countries. *Vaccine* 2016; 34: 5984–9, www.sciencedirect.com/science/article/pii/S0264410X16308568?via%3Dihub.

HPV vaccine statistics: Bruni L et al. Global disparities in HPV vaccination. *Lancet Global Health* 2016; 4: e453-e463, www.thelancet.com/journals/langlo/article/PIIS2214-109X(16)30107-3/fulltext.

Helicobacter pylori: Warren JR, Marshall B. Unidentified curved bacilli on gastric epithelium in active chronic gastritis. *Lancet* 1983; 321: 1273–5.

BCG vaccine and bladder cancer: Chou R et al. Intravesical therapy for the treatment of non-muscle invasive bladder cancer: a systematic review and meta-analysis. *J Urol* 2017; 197: 1189–99.

Sipuleucel-T: Kantoff PW et al. Sipuleucel-T immunotherapy for castration-resistant prostate cancer. *N Engl J Med* 2010; 363: 411–22, www.nejm.org/doi/full/10.1056/NEJMoa1001294.

CHAPTER 9: Vaccines and pregnancy

Riley Hughes: Stein S. Riley Hughes: parents of newborn who died from whooping cough release video of his final moments. ABC News, 14 January 2016, www.abc.net.au/news/2016–01–14/parents-share-video-of-baby-rileys-final-moments/7087434.

Neonatal tetanus on St Kilda: Woody RC, Ross EM. Neonatal tetanus (St Kilda, 19th century). *Lancet* 1989; i: 1339, www.sciencedirect.com/science/article/pii/S014067368992744X.

Maternal and neonatal tetanus statistics: Thwaites CL et al. Maternal and neonatal tetanus. *Lancet* 2015; 385: 362–70; Maternal and neonatal tetanus elimination (MNTE). *World Health Organization*, www.who. int/immunization/diseases/MNTE_initiative/en/.

Influenza and heart attack: Barnes M et al. Acute myocardial infarction and influenza: a meta-analysis of case-control studies. *Heart* 2015; 101: 1738–47, heart.bmj.com/content/101/21/1738; Caldeira D et al. Influenza vaccination and prevention of cardiovascular disease mortality. *Lancet* 2018; 391: 427–8, www.thelancet.com/journals/ lancet/article/PIIS0140-6736(18)30143-0/fulltext.

Maternal influenza immunisation: Mertz D et al. Pregnancy as a risk factor for severe outcomes from influenza virus infection: a systematic review and meta-analysis of observational studies. *Vaccine* 2017; 35: 521–8, www.ncbi.nlm.nih.gov/pmc/articles/PMC5359513/; Nunes MC et al. The effects of influenza vaccination during pregnancy on birth outcomes: a systematic review and meta-analysis. *Am J Perinatol* 2016; 33: 1104–14, www.thieme-connect.com/DOI/ DOI?10.1055/s-0036–1586101; Perrett K, Nolan T. Immunization during pregnancy: impact on the infant. *Pediatr Drugs* 2017; 19: 313–24, link.springer.com/article/10.1007%2Fs40272–017–0231–7; Thompson MG et al. Effectiveness of seasonal trivalent influenza vaccine for preventing influenza virus illness among pregnant women: a population-based case-control study during the 2010–2011 and 2011–2012 influenza seasons. *Clin Infect Dis* 2014; 58: 449–57; Zaman K et al. Effectiveness of maternal influenza immunization in mothers and infants. *N Engl J Med* 2008; 359: 1555–64, www.nejm.org/doi/pdf/10.1056/NEJMoa0708630; Madhi SA et al. Influenza vaccination of pregnant women and protection of their infants. *N Engl J Med* 2014; 371: 918–31, www.nejm.org/doi/ pdf/10.1056/NEJMc1412050; Bratton KN et al. Maternal influenza immunization and birth outcomes of stillbirth and spontaneous abortion: a systematic review and meta-analysis. *Clin Infect Dis* 2015; 60: e11–9, academic.oup.com/cid/article-lookup/doi/10.1093/ cid/ciu915.

Influenza vaccine myths: Misconceptions about seasonal flu and flu vaccines. *Centers for Disease Control and Prevention*, www.cdc.gov/flu/about/ qa/misconceptions.htm.

Cocooning: Healy CM et al. Evaluation of the impact of a pertussis cocooning program on infant pertussis infection. *Pediatr Infect Dis J* 2015; 34: 22–6.

Maternal pertussis immunisation: Vitek CR, Pascual FB, Baughman AL, Murphy TV. Increase in deaths from pertussis among young infants in the United States in the 1990s. *Pediatr Infect Dis J* 2003; 22: 628–634. Amirthalingam G et al. Effectiveness of maternal pertussis vaccination in England: an observational study. *Lancet* 2014; 384: 1521–8; Amirthalingam G et al. Sustained effectiveness of the maternal pertussis immunization program in England 3 years following introduction. *Clin Infect Dis* 2016; 63(Suppl 4): S236–43; Dabrera G et al. A case-control study to estimate the effectiveness of maternal pertussis vaccination in protecting newborn infants in England and Wales, 2012–2013. *Clin Infect Dis* 2015; 60: 333–7.

Norman Gregg: Lancaster PAL. Gregg, Sir Norman McAlister (1892–1966). *Australian Dictionary of Biography*, adb.anu.edu.au/biography/gregg-sir-norman-mcalister-10362; Gregg NM. Congenital cataract following German measles in the mother. *Trans Ophthalmol Soc Austr* 1942; 3: 35–46.

Maternal rubella immunisation: Plotkin SA. The history of rubella and rubella vaccination leading to elimination. *Clin Infect Dis* 2006; 43(Suppl 3): S164–8, academic.oup.com/cid/article/43/Supplement_3/S164/288915; Rubella in the US. *Centers for Disease Control and Prevention*. www.cdc.gov/rubella/about/in-the-us.html; Keller-Stanislawski B et al. Safety of immunization during pregnancy: a review of the evidence of selected inactivated and live attenuated vaccines. *Vaccine* 2014; 32: 7057–64; DeSilva M et al. Congenital anomalies: case definition and guidelines for data collection, analysis, and presentation of immunization safety data. *Vaccine* 2016; 34: 6015–26, www.ncbi.nlm.nih.gov/pmc/articles/PMC5139892/.

CHAPTER 10: Vaccines for the elderly

Shingles and the elderly: Thomas SL et al. Contacts with varicella or with children and protection against herpes zoster in adults: a case-control study. *Lancet* 2002; 360: 678–82, www.thelancet.com/pdfs/journals/lancet/PIIS0140–6736(02)09837–9.pdf; Chapman RS et al.

The incidence of shingles and its implications for vaccination policy. *Vaccine* 2003; 21: 2541–7.

Shingles statistics: McIntyre R et al. Increasing trends of herpes zoster in Australia. *PLoS One* 2015; 10: e0125025; Brisson M et al. Exposure to varicella boosts immunity to herpes-zoster: implications for mass vaccination against chickenpox. *Vaccine* 2002; 20: 2500–7, www.sciencedirect.com/science/article/pii/S0264410X02001809?via%3Dihub; Kawai K et al. Increasing incidence of herpes zoster over a 60-year period from a population-based study. *Clin Infect Dis* 2016; 63: 221–6, www.ncbi.nlm.nih.gov/pmc/articles/PMC4928389/.

Shingles vaccines: Gagliardi AMZ et al. Vaccines for preventing herpes zoster in older adults. *Cochrane Database Syst Rev* 2016, 3: CD008858, cochranelibrary-wiley.com/doi/10.1002/14651858.CD008858.pub3/pdf; Grupping K et al. Immunogenicity and safety of the HZ/su adjuvanted herpes zoster subunit vaccine in adults previously vaccinated with a live attenuated herpes zoster vaccine. *J Infect Dis* 2017; 216: 1343–51, www.ncbi.nlm.nih.gov/pmc/articles/PMC5853346/; Amirthalingam G et al. Evaluation of the effect of the herpes zoster vaccination programme 3 years after its introduction in England: a population-based study. *Lancet Public Health* 2018; 3: e82-e90, www.thelancet.com/journals/lanpub/article/PIIS2468–2667(17)30234–7/fulltext.

Influenza and the elderly: Darvishian M et al. Effectiveness of seasonal influenza vaccination in community-dwelling elderly people: an individual participant data meta-analysis of test-negative design case-control studies. *Lancet Respir Med* 2017; 5: 200–11, www.sciencedirect.com/science/article/pii/S2213260017300437.

CHAPTER 11: The tragedies and the frauds

History of vaccine tragedies: Vaccine timeline. *Immunization Action Coalition,* www.immunize.org/timeline/; Bren L. The road to the biotech revolution: highlights of 100 years of biologics regulation, FDA 2006, *United States Food and Drug Administration,* www.fda.gov/downloads/AboutFDA/WhatWeDo/History/ProductRegulation/UCM593490.pdf.

St Louis tragedy: DeHovitz RE. The 1901 St Louis incident: the first modern medical disaster. *Pediatrics* 2014; 133: 964, pediatrics. aappublications.org/content/133/6/964.full.pdf

Lübeck tragedy: Fox GJ, Orlova M, Schurr E. Tuberculosis in newborns: the lessons of the 'Lübeck disaster' (1929–1933). *PLoS Pathog* 2016; 12: e1005271, journals.plos.org/plospathogens/article?id=10.1371/journal. ppat.1005271.

Bundaberg tragedy: Akers HF, Porter SAT. Bundaberg's Gethsemane: the tragedy of the inoculated children. *RHSQ* 2008; 20: 7, espace.library. uq.edu.au/data/UQ:152716/UQ_PV_152716.pdf; Immunisation inoculation proves fatal: twelve local children die after treatment on Friday. *Bundaberg Daily News and Mail*, 30 January 1928, www. halenet.com.au/~jvbryant/Bundseru.html.

South Sudan tragedy: Fortin J. Mishandled measles vaccine kills 15 children in South Sudan. *New York Times*, 2 June 2017, www.nytimes. com/2017/06/02/international-home/vaccines-south-sudan.html.

Thiomersal: Baker JP. Mercury, vaccines and autism: one controversy, three histories. *Am J Public Health* 2008; 98: 244–53, www.ncbi.nlm.nih. gov/pmc/articles/PMC2376879/.

Aluminium: Mitkus RJ et al. Updated aluminum pharmacokinetics following infant exposures through diet and vaccination. *Vaccine* 2011; 29: 9538–43, www.sciencedirect.com/science/article/pii/ S0264410X11015799?via%3Dihub; Jefferson T, Rudin M, Di Pietrantonj C. Adverse events after immunisation with aluminium-containing DTP vaccines: systematic review of the evidence. *Lancet Infectious Diseases* 2004; 4: 84–90, www.sciencedirect.com/science/ article/pii/S1473309904009272?via%3Dihub.

New adjuvants: Stassinjs J et al. A systematic review and meta-analysis on the safety of newly adjuvanted vaccines among children. *Vaccine* 2016; 34: 714–22, www.sciencedirect.com/science/article/pii/ S0264410X1501796X?via%3Dihub.

Yellow fever: Frierson JG. The yellow fever vaccine: a history. *Yale J Biol Med* 2010; 83: 77–85, www.ncbi.nlm.nih.gov/pmc/articles/PMC2892770/; Emergencies preparedness, response: yellow fever. *World Health Organization*, www.who.int/csr/disease/yellowfev/en/.

Cutter Incident: Offit P. *The Cutter Incident: How America's First Polio Vaccine Led to the Growing Vaccine Crisis.* New Haven: Yale University Press, 2005; Goldacre B. *Bad Pharma: How Drug Companies Mislead Doctors and Harm Patients.* London: 4th Estate, 2012; Langmuir A, Nathanson N, Hall WJ. *The Wyeth Problem: An Epidemiological Analysis of the Occurrence of Poliomyelitis in Association with Certain Lots of the Wyeth Vaccine.* Poliomyelitis Surveillance Unit, Epidemiology Branch, Communicable Diseases Center, Department of Health, Education and Welfare, 1955; Bazin H. *Vaccination: A History from Lady Montagu to Genetic Engineering.* Esher, Surrey: John Libbey Eurotext, 2011; Oshinsky D. *Polio: An American Story.* Oxford: Oxford University Press, 2005.

Andrew Wakefield: Wakefield AJ, Murch SH, Anthony A et al. Ileal lymphoid nodular hyperplasia, non-specific colitis, and pervasive developmental disorder in children (retracted). *Lancet* 1998; 351: 637–41; Elliman D, Bedford H. Hear the silence. *BMJ* 2003; 327: 1411; Deer B. Andrew Wakefield – the fraud investigation. *Brian Deer Award-Winning Investigations*, briandeer.com/mmr/lancet-summary.htm; Godlee F. Wakefield's article linking MMR vaccine and autism was fraudulent. *BMJ* 2011; 342: c7452, www.bmj.com/content/342/bmj.c7452; Ruling on doctor in MMR scare. *NHS*, 29 January 2010, www.nhs.uk/news/medical-practice/ruling-on-doctor-in-mmr-scare/; Murch SH, Anthony A et al. Retraction of an interpretation. *Lancet* 2004; 363: 750; Deer B. How the case against the MMR vaccine was fixed. *BMJ* 2011; 342: c5347, www.bmj.com/content/342/bmj.c5347; Deer B. How the vaccine crisis was meant to make money. *BMJ* 2011; 342: c5258, www.bmj.com/content/342/bmj.c5258; Deer B. Wakefield accused of fraud in US trial. *Brian Deer Award-Winning Investigations*, briandeer.com/solved/cedillo-wakefield.htm; Glenza J. Disgraced anti-vaxxer Andrew Wakefield aims to advance his agenda in Texas election. *Guardian*, 26 February 2018, www.theguardian.com/us-news/2018/feb/26/texas-vaccinations-safety-andrew-wakefield-fear-elections.

John Walker-Smith: *Walker-Smith v General Medical Council.* [2012] EWHC 503 (Admin) Case No: CO/7039/2010; Dyer C. Co-author of Wakefield paper on MMR vaccine wins his appeal against decision

by GMC to strike him off. *BMJ* 20122; 344: e1745, www.bmj.com/
content/344/bmj.e1745.

Measles mmunisation rates: Measles notifications and deaths in England
and Wales: 1940 to 2016. *Public Health England*. www.gov.uk/
government/publications/measles-deaths-by-age-group-from-1980-
to-2013-ons-data/measles-notifications-and-deaths-in-england-and-
wales-1940-to-2013; McBrien J et al. Measles outbreak in Dublin,
2000. *Pediatr Infect Dis J* 2003; 22: 580–4; Zelinski A. Number
of unvaccinated children has soared. *Houston Chronicle*, 13 April
2017, www.houstonchronicle.com/news/local/article/Number-of-un-
vaccinated-children-has-soared-11071051.php.

Rotavirus: Soares-Weiser K et al. Vaccines for preventing rotavirus diarrhoea:
vaccines in use. *Cochrane Database Syst Rev* 2012: 11; CD008521;
Australian Government Department of Health. *The Australian
Immunisation Handbook*. 10th ed. Canberra: Commonwealth of
Australia, 2015, 4.17.11, Rotavirus, Adverse effects, www.immunise.
health.gov.au/internet/immunise/publishing.nsf/Content/Handbook10-
home~handbook10part4~handbook10–4-17#4.17.11; Kassim P,
Eslick GD. Risk of intussusception following rotavirus vaccination:
an evidence based meta-analysis of cohort and case-control studies.
Vaccine 2017; 35: 4276–86.

OPV versus IPV: Tucker AW et al. Cost-effectiveness analysis of changing
from live oral poliovirus vaccine to inactivated poliovirus vaccine in
Australia. *Aust NZ J Public Health* 2001; 25:411–6.

CHAPTER 12: The modern anti-immunisation movement

Jenny McCarthy: Offit P. *Autism's False Prophets: Bad Medicine, Risky
Medicine, and the Search for a Cure*. Columbia: Columbia University
Press, 2008.

MMR immunisation in the United States: National Center for Health
Statistics: immunization. *Centers for Disease Control and Prevention*,
www.cdc.gov/nchs/fastats/immunize.htm.

Andrew Wakefield in the United States: Whipple, T. Who is Andrew Wakefield
and what's his link to Donald Trump? *The Times*, 8 May 2017.

Donald Trump: Trump DJ. Tweet, 28 March 2014, twitter.com/
realdonaldtrump/status/449525268529815552?lang=en; Freedman A.

Trump decries 'tremendous increase' in US autism cases. But it's not so simple. *Mashable*, 15 February 2017, www.yahoo.com/news/trump-decries-tremendous-increase-u-221230113.html.

Autism: Kanner L. Autistic disturbances of affective contact. *Nervous Child* 1943; 2: 217–250.

George Bernard Shaw: Shaw GB. *The Doctor's Dilemma, Getting Married, and the Shewing-Up of Blanco Posnet.* New York: Brentano's, 1911.

Julie Leask: Attwell K, Leask J et al. Vaccine rejecting parents' engagement with expert systems that inform vaccination programs. *Bioethical Enquiry* 2017; 14: 65, link.springer.com/article/10.1007/s11673–016–9756–7; Leask J et al. Should we do battle with antivaccination activists? *Public Health Res Pract* 2015; 25: e2521515, www.phrp.com.au/issues/march-2015-volume-25-issue-2/should-we-do-battle-with-antivaccination-activists; Dunn AG, Surian D, Leask J et al. Mapping information exposure on social media to explain differences in HPV vaccine coverage in the United States. *Vaccine* 2017; 35: 3033–40, www.sciencedirect.com/science/article/pii/S0264410X17305522.

Pru Hobson-West: Hobson-West P. 'Trusting blindly can be the biggest risk of all': organised resistance to childhood vaccination in the United Kingdom. *Sociol Health Illn* 2007; 29: 198–215, dx.doi.org/10.1111/j.1467–9566.2007.00544.x.

Vaccines and immune system stimulation: Higgins JPT et al. Association of BCG, DTP, and measles containing vaccines with childhood mortality: systematic review. *BMJ* 2016; 355: i5170, www.bmj.com/content/355/bmj.i5170.long; Kandasamy R et al. Non-specific immunological effects of selected routine childhood immunisations: systematic review. *BMJ* 2016; 355: i5225, www.bmj.com/content/355/bmj.i5225

HPV immunisation in Japan: Hanley SJ et al. HPV vaccination crisis in Japan. *Lancet* 2015; 385: 2571.

HPV immunisation in France: Lefèvre H et al. HPV vaccination rate in French adolescent girls: an example of vaccine distrust. *Arch Dis Child* 2018; 103: 740–6, adc.bmj.com/content/103/8/740.

HPV immunisation in the United States: Udesky L. Push to mandate HPV vaccine triggers backlash in USA. *Lancet* 2007; 369: 979–80; Knox R. HPV vaccine: the science behind the controversy. *NPR*, 19 September

2011, www.npr.org/2011/09/19/140543977/hpv-vaccine-the-science-behind-the-controversy; National Center for Health Statistics: immunization. *Centers for Disease Control and Prevention*, www.cdc.gov/nchs/fastats/immunize.htm.

HPV immunisation in Australia: Coverage data. *National HPV Vaccination Program Register*, www.hpvregister.org.au/research/coverage-data.

Katie Couric: Jaslow R. Katie Couric admits disproportionate reporting on HPV vaccine controversy. *CBS News*, 10 December 2013, www.cbsnews.com/news/katie-couric-hpv-vaccine-show-criticism-valid/; Couric K. Furthering the conversation on the HPV vaccine. *Huffpost*, 10 December 2013, www.huffingtonpost.com/katie-couric/vaccine-hpv-furthering-conversation_b_4418568.html?1386687305.

Merck: Tomljenovic L, Shaw CA. Too fast or not too fast: the FDA's approval of Merck's HPV vaccine Gardasil. *J Law Med Ethics* 2012; 40: 673–81.

Trust: Birkhäue J et al. Trust in the healthcare professional and health outcome: a meta-analysis. *PLoS One* 2017; 12: e0170988, www.ncbi.nlm.nih.gov/pmc/articles/PMC5295692/pdf/pone.0170988.pdf.

Hepatitis B immunisation in France: Ascherio A et al. Hepatitis B vaccination and the risk of multiple sclerosis. *N Engl J Med* 2001; 344: 327–32; Le Houézec D. Evolution of multiple sclerosis in France since the beginning of hepatitis B vaccination. *Immunol Res.* 2014; 60: 219-25, www.ncbi.nlm.nih.gov/pmc/articles/PMC4266455/.

CHAPTER 13: Immunisation and ethics

Hippocrates: Lloyd GER (ed), Chadwick J (transl). *Hippocratic Writings*. London: Penguin Classics, 1950.

Bioethics: Kerridge I, Lowe M, Stewart C. *Ethics, Law and the Health Profession*. 4th ed. Sydney: Federation Press, 2013.

Nazi doctors: Annas GJ, Grodin MA (eds). *The Nazi Doctors and the Nuremberg Code*. New York: Oxford University Press, 1992.

Tuskegee Study: Jones JH. *Bad Blood: The Tuskegee Syphilis Experiment*. New York: The Free Press, 1993; US Public Health Service syphilis study at Tuskegee: presidential apology. *Centers for Disease Control and Prevention*, 16 May 1997, www.cdc.gov/tuskegee/clintonp.htm.

Willowbrook experiments: Fansiwala K. The duality of medicine: the Willowbrook State School experiments. *The Review & Debates*, 20 February 2016, www.thereviewatnyu.com/all/2016/2/20/the-duality-of-medicine-the-willowbrook-state-school-experiments.

Vaccines developed from aborted foetuses: Luño AR. Ethical reflections on vaccines using cells from aborted foetuses. *National Catholic Bioethics Quarterly* 2006; 6: 453–9, www.ncbcenter.org/index.php/download_file/force/178/159/; Vatican statement on vaccines derived from aborted human foetuses. *Immunization Action Coalition*, www.immunize.org/concerns/vaticandocument.htm.

Tom Beauchamp and Jim Childress: Beauchamp TL, Childress JF. *Principles of Biomedical Ethics*. New York: Oxford University Press, 1977.

John Stuart Mill: Mill JS. *On Liberty*. London: John W Parker & Son, 1859, ebooks.adelaide.edu.au/m/mill/john_stuart/m645o/index.html.

Hepatitis B intervention: Isaacs D. Children have rights, too. *J Paediatr Child Health* 2009; 45: 627–8, onlinelibrary.wiley.com/doi/10.1111/j.1440–1754.2009.01620.x/full; Isaacs D et al. Ethical issues in preventing mother-to-child transmission of hepatitis B by immunisation. *Vaccine* 2011; 29: 6159–62.

Rabies interventions: Hampson K et al. Rabies exposures, post-exposure prophylaxis and deaths in a region of endemic canine rabies. *PLoS Negl Trop Dis* 2008; 2: e339, www.ncbi.nlm.nih.gov/pmc/articles/PMC2582685/.

2017 European measles outbreaks: Measles continues to spread and take lives in Europe. *World Health Organization, Regional Office for Europe*, 11 July 2017, www.euro.who.int/en/media-centre/sections/press-releases/2017/measles-continues-to-spread-and-take-lives-in-europe; Measles outbreaks still ongoing in 2018 and fatalities reported from four countries. *European Centre for Disease Prevention and Control*, 9 March 2018, ecdc.europa.eu/en/news-events/measles-outbreaks-still-ongoing-2018-and-fatalities-reported-four-countries.

Belgium polio case: Stafford N. Belgian parents are sentenced to prison for not vaccinating children. *BMJ* 2008; 336: 348, www.bmj.com/content/336/7640/348.1.full.

No Jab No Play/Pay: No Jab No Play, No Jab No Pay policies. *National Centre for Immunisation Research & Surveillance*, www.ncirs.edu.au/consumer-resources/no-jab-no-play-no-jab-no-pay-policies/.

Northern New South Wales tetanus case: MacKenzie B. Vaccination debate flares on NSW north coast after 7yo contracts tetanus. *ABC News*, 16 March 2017,www.abc.net.au/news/2017–03–17/tetanus-girl-not-vaccinated-say-health-authorities/8362722.

Indiana hospital case: Lupkin S. Eight hospital employees fired for refusing flu vaccines. *ABC News* (United States), 3 January 2012, abcnews.go.com/Health/indiana-hospital-fires-nurses-refusing-flu-shot/story?id=18116967.

Vaccine injury compensation schemes: National Vaccine Injury Compensation Program. *Health Resources & Services Administration*, www.hrsa.gov/vaccine-compensation/index.html; Looker C, Kelly H. No-fault compensation following adverse events attributed to vaccination: a review of international programmes. *Bull WHO* 2011; 89: 371–8, www.ncbi.nlm.nih.gov/pmc/articles/PMC3089384/; Isaacs D. Should Australia introduce a vaccine injury compensation scheme? *J Paediatr Child Health* 2004; 40: 247–9.

CHAPTER 14: Overcoming the iniquity of poverty

Immunisation statistics: Immunization. *World Health Organization*, www.who.int/topics/immunization/en/.

WHO Expanded Programme on Immunization: The immunization programme that saved millions of lives. *Bull WHO* 2014; 92: 314–5, www.who.int/bulletin/volumes/92/5/14–020514/en/.

Halfdan Mahler: De Leeuw E. A tribute to Dr Halfdan Mahler, 1923–2016. *Health Prom Int* 2017; 32: 1, academic.oup.com/heapro/article/32/1/1/2964736.

UNICEF: Adamson P et al. *Jim Grant: UNICEF Visionary*. Geneva: UNICEF Innocenti Research Centre, 2001, www.unicef.org/french/publications/files/Jim-Grant-LR.pdf; United Nations Children's Fund, World Health Organization. *Immunization Summary: A Statistical Reference Containing Data Through 2011*. New York: United Nations Children's Fund, 2012, www.unicef.org/immunization/files/EN-ImmSumm-2013.pdf;UNICEF people: Danny Kaye. *UNICEF*, www.unicef.org/people/people_danny_kaye.html.

March of Dimes: Rose D. A history of the March of Dimes, *March of Dimes*, 26 August 2010, www.marchofdimes.org/mission/a-history-of-the-march-of-dimes.aspx.

Rotary: Our foundation. *Rotary*, www.rotary.org/en/about-rotary/rotary-foundation; You've probably never heard of Clem Renouf – but his idea changed the world. *I Boost Immunity*, iboostimmunity.com/articles/youve-probably-never-heard-clem-renouf-his-idea-changed-world; End polio. *Rotary*, my.rotary.org/en/take-action/end-polio.

Bill and Melinda Gates: *Bill & Melinda Gates Foundation*, www.gatesfoundation.org/; *Gavi, the Vaccine Alliance*, www.gavi.org/.

HPV immunisation: Millions of girls in developing countries to be protected against cervical cancer thanks to new HPV vaccine deals. *Gavi, The Vaccine Alliance*, 9 May 2013, www.gavi.org/library/news/press-releases/2013/hpv-price-announcement/; Gallagher KE et al. Status of HPV vaccine introduction and barriers to country uptake. *Vaccine* 2018; 36: 4761–7, www.sciencedirect.com/science/article/pii/S0264410X18301671?via%3Dihub.

Hepatitis B immunisation: Hepatitis B, *World Health Organization*, www.who.int/immunization/diseases/hepatitisB/en/.

Measles immunisation: Measles, *World Health Organization*, www.who.int/immunization/diseases/measles/en/.

Cameron government: Heppell T, Lightfoot S. 'We will not balance the books on the backs of the poorest people in the world': understanding Conservative Party strategy on international aid. *Political Q* 2012; 83: 130–8; Cameron D. David Cameron: why we're right to ringfence the aid budget. *Guardian*, 12 June 2011,www.theguardian.com/global-development/2011/jun/11/david-cameron-defends-aid-funding.

Paul Wilson report: Wilson P. *Giving Developing Countries the Best Shot: An Overview of Vaccine Access and R&D*. Oxfam International, Médecins Sans Frontières, 2010, www.oxfam.org/sites/www.oxfam.org/files/giving-developing-countries-best-shot-vaccines-2010–05.pdf.

Meningococcal C vaccine: Trotter CL et al. Effectiveness of meningococcal serogroup C conjugate vaccine 4 years after introduction. *Lancet* 2004; 364: 365–7, www.thelancet.com/journals/lancet/article/PIIS0140–6736(04)16725–1/fulltext.

PATH: Better health moves humanity forward. *PATH*, www.path.org/about/
   index.php.
Meningitis Vaccine Project: Kiffay T et al. The evolution of the Meningitis
   Vaccine Project. *Clin Infect Dis* 2015; 61 (Suppl 5): S396–403, www.
   ncbi.nlm.nih.gov/pmc/articles/PMC4639496/.
Meningococcal A immunisation in Chad: Daugla DM et al. Effect of a
   serogroup A meningococcal conjugate vaccine (PsA–TT) on serogroup
   A meningococcal meningitis and carriage in Chad: a community
   study. *Lancet* 2014; 383: 40–7, www.thelancet.com/journals/lancet/
   article/PIIS0140–6736(13)61612–8/fulltext.
Immunisation coverage: Immunization coverage. *World Health Organisation*,
   www.who.int/mediacentre/factsheets/fs378/en/.

CHAPTER 15: Immunisation into the future

Top 10 causes of death: The top 10 causes of death. *World Health
   Organization*, www.who.int/en/news-room/fact-sheets/detail/the-top-
   10-causes-of-death.
Effective use of vaccines: *Investing in Immunisation Through the GAVI
   Alliance: The Evidence Base*, Geneva: GAVI Alliance, 2012,
   www.gavi.org/library/publications/the-evidence-base/investing-in-
   immunisation-through-the-gavi-alliance---the-evidence-base/.
Malaria: Gomes PS et al. Immune escape strategies of malaria parasites.
   Front Microbiol 2016; 7: 1617,www.ncbi.nlm.nih.gov/pmc/articles/
   PMC5066453/.
HIV: Naughtie A. HIV 'invisibility cloak' allows virus to evade immune
   system. *The Conversation*, 7 November 2013, theconversation.
   com/hiv-invisibility-cloak-allows-virus-to-evade-immune-
   system-19918; Understanding how HIV evades the immune
   system. *Science Daily*, 21 February 2017, www.sciencedaily.com/
   releases/2017/02/170221110654.htm.
Malaria statistics: Malaria. *World Health Organization*, www.who.int/
   malaria/en/.
HIV statistics: HIV. *World Health Organization*, www.who.int/hiv/en/.
Dementia statistics: *Dementia: A Public Health Priority*. Geneva: World
   Health Organization, Alzheimer's Disease International, 2012, www.
   who.int/mental_health/neurology/dementia/en/.

Dementia vaccines: Marciani DJ. A retrospective analysis of the Alzheimer's disease vaccine progress – the critical need for new development strategies. *J Neurochem* 2016; 137: 687–700, onlinelibrary.wiley.com/doi/10.1111/jnc.13608/epdf; Pasquier F et al. Two phase 2 multiple ascending-dose studies of vanutide cridificar (ACC-001) and QS-21 adjuvant in mild-to-moderate Alzheimer's disease. *J Alzheimers Dis* 2016; 51: 1131–43, content.iospress.com/articles/journal-of-alzheimers-disease/jad150376; Novak P et al. Safety and immunogenicity of the tau vaccine AADvac1 in patients with Alzheimer's disease: a randomised, double-blind, placebo-controlled, phase 1 trial. *Lancet Neurol* 2017; 16: 123–34, www.sciencedirect.com/science/article/pii/S1474442216303313?via%3Dihub.

Helicobacter pylori: Ming Z et al. Efficacy, safety, and immunogenicity of an oral recombinant *Helicobacter pylori* vaccine in children in China: a randomised, double-blind, placebo-controlled, phase 3 trial. *Lancet* 2015; 386: 1457–64, www.thelancet.com/pdfs/journals/lancet/PIIS0140–6736(15)60310–5.pdf; Muljono DH. In conversation with Barry Marshall: using pathogens to help humans. *The Conversation*, 30 March 2016, theconversation.com/in-conversation-with-barry-marshall-using-pathogens-to-help-humans-56153.

Edible vaccines: Concha C et al. Disease prevention: an opportunity to expand edible plant-based vaccines? *Vaccines (Basel)* 2017; 5: 14, ncbi.nlm.nih.gov/pmc/articles/PMC5492011/.

Nasal RSV vaccine: Neuzil KM. Progress toward a respiratory syncytial virus vaccine. *Clin Vaccine Immunol* 2016; 23: 186–8, cvi.asm.org/content/23/3/186.full.

Jet injectors: Resik S et al. Needle-free jet injector intradermal delivery of fractional dose inactivated poliovirus vaccine: association between injection quality and immunogenicity. *Vaccine* 2015; 33: 5873–7, www.sciencedirect.com/science/article/pii/S0264410X15008725?via%3Dihub; Jackson L et al. Safety and immunogenicity of varying dosages of trivalent inactivated influenza vaccine administered by needle-free jet injectors. *Vaccine* 2001; 19: 4703–9, www.sciencedirect.com/science/article/pii/S0264410X01002250?via%3Dihub; Canter J et al. An outbreak of hepatitis B associated with jet injections in a weight reduction clinic.

Arch Internal Med 1990; 150: 1923–7, jamanetwork.com/journals/
jamainternalmedicine/article-abstract/613868.

Microneedles: Pearson FE et al. Functional anti-polysaccharide IgG
titres induced by unadjuvanted pneumococcal-conjugate vaccine
when delivered by microprojection-based skin patch. *Vaccine*
2015; 33: 6675–83, www.sciencedirect.com/science/article/pii/
S0264410X15015248?via%3Dihub; Van der Maaden K et al.
Microneedle technologies for (trans)dermal drug and vaccine
delivery. *J Control Release* 2012; 161: 645–55, www.sciencedirect.
com/science/article/pii/S0168365912000740?via%3Dihub; Raphael
AP et al. Formulations for microprojection/microneedle vaccine
delivery: structure, strength and release profiles *J Control Release*
2016; 225: 40–52, www.sciencedirect.com/science/article/pii/
S0168365916300220?via%3Dihub; Rouphael NG et al. The safety,
immunogenicity, and acceptability of inactivated influenza vaccine
delivered by microneedle patch (TIV-MNP 2015): a randomised,
partly blinded, placebo-controlled, phase 1 trial. *Lancet* 2017; 390:
649–58, www.thelancet.com/journals/lancet/article/PIIS0140-
6736(17)30575-5/fulltext.

Glossary of terms and abbreviations

Adjuvant A substance added to a vaccine to improve the immune response.

ADT The name of an adult diphtheria and tetanus vaccine, used as a 'booster' for previously immunised adults and children over five.

AEFI Adverse events following immunisation; this term is preferred to calling them vaccine side effects, because they may have been caused by the vaccine or may have occurred by coincidence.

Antibiotics Substances that destroy bacteria and are used to treat bacterial infections.

Antibodies Proteins produced by the immune system in response to antigens. The antigens may come from an organism causing an infection or from a vaccine. Another name for an antibody is an immunoglobulin.

Antigens Foreign substances that stimulate an immune response.

Attenuated An attenuated vaccine has been modified so it is still alive but is harmless or unlikely to cause a severe infection. Examples are viral vaccines like measles, mumps and rubella (MMR), chickenpox and rotavirus vaccines, and the bacterial BCG vaccine against tuberculosis.

BCG Bacille Calmette–Guérin vaccine against tuberculosis, a live attenuated vaccine, and the oldest vaccine still in use.

CDC Centers for Disease Control, the United States national health protection agency

Conjugate vaccines Highly effective vaccines produced by joining (conjugating) outer-coat polysaccharides (which do not stimulate an immune response in infants) to a protein that does elicit an immune response, in order to generate better immunity, e.g. Hib, meningococcal and pneumococcal conjugate vaccines.

DT The general abbreviation for childhood diphtheria and tetanus vaccines, the capital letters indicating higher concentrations of the diphtheria toxoid.

dT The general abbreviation for adult diphtheria and tetanus vaccines, which have lower levels of the diphtheria toxoid than childhood preparations.

DTPa A three-in-one diphtheria, tetanus and pertussis vaccine. The small 'a' indicates acellular pertussis vaccine, a more purified form.

dTpa An adult three-in-one diphtheria, tetanus and pertussis vaccine with lower levels of antigens than DTPa. Used for pregnant women.

DTPw A three-in-one diphtheria, tetanus and pertussis vaccine. The small 'w' indicates whole-cell pertussis vaccine, containing inactivated whole pertussis bacteria.

Encephalitis Inflammation of the brain.

Endemic An endemic infection is one that is always present in a community, e.g. malaria is endemic in most of Africa.

Epidemic A rapidly spreading outbreak of infection, e.g. influenza epidemics occur every winter but disappear in summer.

FDA   The Food and Drug Administration, an agency of the United States Health Department that oversees the safety of foods, drugs and vaccines.

Gastroenteritis   An illness characterised by diarrhoea, often with vomiting and abdominal pain, Mostly caused by viruses, e.g. rotaviruses and noroviruses. Often known as 'gastro'.

Gavi   Gavi, the Vaccine Alliance, previously the Global Alliance for Vaccines and Immunization (GAVI), is a partnership to promote immunisation in poor countries. It was started in 2000, and has received massive financial support from the Bill and Melinda Gates Foundation.

Haemophilus influenzae type b   See Hib.

Hepatitis   Inflammation of the liver.

Hib   An abbreviation of *Haemophilus influenzae* type b, an organism that can cause bloodstream infection and meningitis in infants and young children. There are highly effective vaccines available.

HPV   Human papillomavirus, a virus that can cause a range of diseases, including cervical cancer.

Immune response   The body's protective mechanism against disease.

Immunisation   The process of giving a vaccine to induce immunity or protection from infection (often used interchangeably with 'vaccination').

Immunity   Protection from infection.

Infection   When an organism enters the body; infection can be asymptomatic (latent) or can cause a symptomatic illness.

Intussusception   Telescoping of an infant's bowel, blocking it and requiring treatment or even an operation. Can occur spontaneously and is a very rare complication of rotavirus vaccines.

IPV   Inactivated polio vaccine.

Meningococcus Another name for a bacterium called *Neisseria meningitidis* that can cause serious meningococcal infections, including bloodstream infection and meningitis, at any age, but particularly in infants and young adults. There are frequent severe epidemics in sub-Saharan Africa. There are highly effective vaccines available.

MMR Measles-mumps-rubella vaccine.

OPV Oral polio vaccine.

Pandemic A global epidemic, almost always of influenza. The most recent was the 'swine flu' pandemic of 2009.

Pneumococcus Another name for a bacterium called *Streptococcus pneumoniae* that can cause serious infections, including pneumonia and meningitis, particularly in infants and the elderly. Aboriginal people and Native Americans have a high incidence of pneumococcal infections. There are highly effective vaccines available.

Polysaccharide vaccines Vaccines made from purified polysaccharides (sugars) in the outer capsule of bacteria, e.g. pneumococcal polysaccharide vaccine.

RCT Randomised controlled trial, a scientific study in which patients are assigned at random to one or another treatment, minimising bias. In a 'double-blind' RCT, neither the patient nor the doctor knows which treatment the patient received.

Shingles Colloquial term for zoster.

Toxins Harmful substances produced by bacteria, e.g. *Corynebacterium diphtheriae* toxin causes the worst symptoms of diphtheria, and *Clostridium tetani* toxin causes the muscle spasms of tetanus.

Toxoid vaccines Vaccines produced by treating bacterial toxins so that they are no longer harmful but stimulate an immune response, e.g. diphtheria toxoid, tetanus toxoid.

Vaccination   The process of giving a vaccine (often used interchangeably with 'immunisation').

Vaccine   A biological substance manufactured to produce immunity to an infectious organism.

Varicella zoster virus (VZV)   Chickenpox virus. After people recover from chickenpox, the virus remains in their nerves and can reactivate years later as zoster (shingles). There are live attenuated chickenpox vaccines.

Virus   A minuscule infectious organism, 1000 times smaller than a human cell, that needs to reproduce in cells.

WHO   The World Health Organization, a subsidiary of the United Nations, established in 1948 and based in Geneva.

Zoster   A painful rash on one side of the body or face caused by reactivation of infection with the chickenpox virus (varicella zoster virus, VZV). Also called shingles. There are live attenuated zoster vaccines.

Suggested reading

Australian Government Department of Health. *The Australian Immunisation Handbook*. 10th ed. Canberra: Commonwealth of Australia, 2015. Updated version available online since December 2017: immunisationhandbook.health.gov.au/.

Australian Government Department of Health and Ageing. *Myths and Realities Responding to Arguments Against Vaccination – A Guide for Providers*. 5th ed. Canberra: Commonwealth of Australia, 2013, beta.health.gov.au/resources/publications/myths-realities-about-immunisation.

Ada G, Isaacs D. *Vaccination: The Facts, the Fears, the Future*. Sydney: Allen & Unwin, 2000.

Offit P. *The Cutter Incident*. New Haven/London: Yale University Press, 2005.

Offit P. *Autism's False Prophets: Bad Medicine, Risky Medicine, and the Search for a Cure*. Columbia: Columbia University Press, 2008.

Offit PA. *Deadly Choices: How the Anti-Vaccine Movement Threatens Us All*. New York: Basic Books, 2010.

Plotkin SA, Orenstein WA, Offit P, Edwards KM (eds). *Vaccines*. 7th ed. Philadelphia: Elsevier Saunders, 2017.

Acknowledgments

My special thanks to Mary Rennie for suggesting I write this book, which I found an exhilarating process. Mary was tirelessly enthusiastic, and kept coming up with new stories for me to investigate and great advice about what to include and what to leave out. I loved doing the reading necessary to learn more, and I learned a lot of things I really ought to have known already. My wonderful colleague Ken Nunn told me that a friend once described him as an encyclopaedia of slightly inaccurate information. This describes me to a tee. I would be embarrassed by my ignorance if embarrassment were still in my armoury.

There are too many people with whom I have discussed immunisation over the years to remember, let alone acknowledge here, but I would particularly like to thank Ross Andrews, Chris Blyth, Robert Booy, Philip Britton, David Burgner, Margaret Burgess, Jim Buttery, David Durrheim, Dominic Dwyer, the late Frank Fenner, Robert Hall, Alyson Kakakios, Sam Katz, Ian Kerridge, Henry Kilham, Simon Kroll, Julie Leask, Mike Levin, Kristine Macartney, Aidan Macfarlane, Peter McIntyre, Jodie McVernon, Ben Marais, Helen Marshall, Sam Mehr, Liz

Miller, Richard Moxon, Terry Nolan, Gus Nossal, Paul Offit, Stan Plotkin, Andrew Pollard, Jenny Royle, David Salisbury and Melanie Wong for the special contributions they have made to my thoughts on all aspects of immunisation. I thank Robert Booy, Phil Britton, Adam Dunn, David Durrheim, Mark Isaacs, Tim Knapp, Julie Leask, John Pearn and Kartika Putra for reading early chapter drafts and making helpful comments.

Mary Rennie and Shannon Kelly from HarperCollins gave me enormous help with my first ham-fisted draft chapters, and I am in total awe of their ability to read a chapter and make incredibly insightful and constructive suggestions. Scott Forbes of HarperCollins proved equally incisive and insightful as the book neared completion. I must express my special thanks to the wonderful Emma Dowden. Emma is a freelance editor who was handed my over-long and over-garrulous manuscript, full as it was of irrelevant and distracting digressions fascinating only to me. Emma sifted the chaff from the grain and reorganised the entire book in a way which still fills me with awe. How did she do that?

Finally, I would like to thank my wife, Carmel, for her selfless support and devotion, and for putting up with me for all the years we have been together. She has been a constant inspiration to me and to our wonderful children. She is the lodestar of my existence. I would be lost without her.

David Isaacs, 2019

Index